MATHEMATICS FORMULAE

Sumita Bose

I0125120

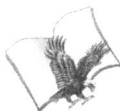

V&S PUBLISHERS

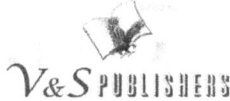

Published by

V&S PUBLISHERS

F-2/16, Ansari Road, Daryaganj, New Delhi-110002
011-23240026, 011-23240027 • *Fax* 011-23240028
Email info@vspublishers.com • *Website* www.vspublishers.com

Regional Office Hyderabad
5-1-707/1, Brij Bhawan (Beside Central Bank of India Lane)
Bank Street, Koti, Hyderabad - 500 095
040-24737290
E-mail vspublishershyd@gmail.com

Branch Office : Mumbai
Jaywant Industrial Estate, 2nd Floor–222, Tardeo Road
Opposite Sobo Central Mall, Mumbai – 400 034
022-23510736
E-mail: vspublishersmum@gmail.com

Follow us on

All books available at **www.vspublishers.com**

© **Copyright :** V&S PUBLISHERS
ISBN 978-93-505719-6-5
Edition 2015

The Copyright of this book, as well as all matter contained herein (including illustrations) rests with the Publisher. No person shall copy the name of the book, its title design, matter and illustrations in any form and in any language, totally or partially or in any form. Anybody doing so shall face legal action and will be responsible for damages.

Printed at Param Offseters Okhla New Delhi-110020

Publisher's Note

After publishing various general trade and mass appeal books, V&S publishers, the fastest growing publisher of India, is pleased to bring out *'Mathematics Formulae'* the book which not only helps in understanding the basics of mathematical concepts but also provides the students with hints to arrive at the solution. To go through an examination successfully, the aspirants need to learn all the formulae and basics covered in the syllabus and increase their efficiency in solving the problems asked in the exams. While attending school and competitive examinations, students need to recollect and apply exact mathematical formulae. A candidate cannot reach the right solution until he/she makes use of the right formula. Therefore, application of the exact formula ensures the right solution and right answer to the question.

This book provides a quick glance at commonly needed formulae for Arithmetic, Algebra, Boolean Algebra, Geometry, Trigonometry, Calculus, Coordinate Geometry, Vectors, Dynamics and Statistics. The book is not only designed for the students and job aspirants but it is also a quick reference and handy guide for the teachers. This book contains relevant definitions to clear basic concepts, useful axioms, theorems and their properties, easy mnemonics for conversion of units, appendix containing mathematical constants, log tables and trigonometric tables. Many practical tips to boost the level of performance, attractive diagrammatic illustrations and usage of simple and lucid language make this book a unique piece of work.

We wish you success in all examinations and a very bright future in the field of mathematics.

Good Luck!!!

Contents

Introduction

Competitive examinations are mainly of two types – *entrance examination (*for admission purpose*)* and *recruitment examination (*for job purpose), whatever be the type, mathematics plays an important role. Like the crest of peacock, mathematics in the name of quantitative aptitude, quantitative ability, numerical ability etc. is at the head of all competitive examinations. This book is a resource help in navigating the labyrinth that is the preparation for competitive examination. The only method to score well in Mathematics is to clear the basic concept and memorize all the formulae followed by regular practice.

My sincere effort is to take away the uncertainty that crops up when a student knows the method of solving a problem but is not able to do so due to lack of remembrance of the associated formulae. This book is divided into different branches of Mathematics for easy navigation. It has comprehensive coverage of **Arithmetic, Algebra, Geometry, Trigonometry, Calculus, Vectors, Coordinate Geometry, Dynamics** and **Statistics** Formulae. This book is not only designed for the students and job aspirants but it is also a quick reference and handy guide for the teachers.

15 Tips to Boost Your Performance

Every student aspires to get admission in a reputed college and every person taking a recruitment examination hopes to get his/her dream job. The following tips will help to go through the competitive examination and score high marks in them.

1. **Set your goal**

   The students should have a clear picture in their mind regarding their objectives and goals. They should make a choice and set their goals to become successful.

2. **Know about prerequisites**

   Prior to the preparation for any examination, the eligibility criteria should be determined. For example:

   (a) Age requirement for the examination

   (b) Required qualification

   (c) Required percentage of marks

3. **Ensure your planning is proper**

   Proper planning lays the foundation stone for any exam preparation. The first part of planning involves the knowledge of the following things:

   (a) Time of the year when the examination form is released

   (b) Number of times a particular examination is held in a year

   (c) Last date for submission of the form

   (d) List of things to be submitted along with the form, for example photographs, mark sheet etc.

   (e) Mode of payment for the examination fee – cheque, draft, credit card etc.

   The second part of the planning involves the knowledge of the examination pattern (stay updated as the syllabus and the examination pattern might change)

   (a) Subjects involved

   (b) Syllabus of each subject

   (c) Time duration of the examination

(d) Number of questions to be attempted

(e) Marking scheme (Check whether negative marking is a part of the scheme)

The third part is the preparation plan. The student has to decide whether he/she wants to join a coaching centre, some online course, study with friends or just do self study.

4. **Utilize all available resources**

   The students must make use of all possible resources. This includes good books, free online material, study material of seniors etc.

5. **Carry out SWOT analysis**

   SWOT stands for

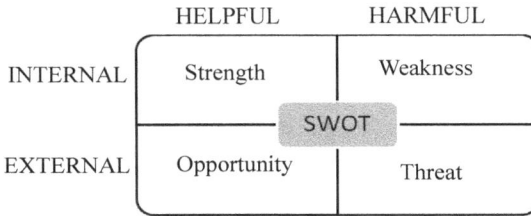

	HELPFUL	HARMFUL
INTERNAL	Strength	Weakness
	SWOT	
EXTERNAL	Opportunity	Threat

Identification of SWOT is important because it can help in improving the plan to achieve the objective. SWOT analysis can help the students to become more focused. Strength and weakness are internal factors whereas opportunity and threat are external factors.

Strength: The students need to identify their strength and enhance them to score well in the competitive examination.

Weakness: Identification of weakness will help the student to overcome it. The students should take professional help to do this if required.

Opportunity: The identification of opportunity will help the students to make the best use of it. For example, the students may exchange books or study material with their friends if possible.

Threat: Identification of threat will help the student to overcome it. For example, if the surrounding environment is too noisy during the afternoon the student can rest in the afternoon and study at night.

6. **Maintain self discipline**

   The preparation should be started well in advance. The students should not get easily diverted by the television shows, social media etc. Regularity is very important for the preparation.

7. **Clear basic concepts**

This is especially important in Mathematics. Many students do not study Mathematics in Class XI, XII/College. As a result they tend to forget the basics. Hence, during preparation the chapters should be started right from the basics.

8. **Keep a positive attitude**

Hellen Keller said, "Optimism is the faith that leads to achievement. Nothing can be done without hope and confidence." Hence, the students must work hard, remain confident and always keep a positive attitude.

9. **Optimize time management**

Time management is about accuracy of choices.

Self Assessment: The students can make a chart for self assessment. This will help in adjusting the time.

Weekly Schedule: The best method of time management is to create a weekly schedule prioritizing the subjects/chapters. At the end of the week it should be evaluated. If the target is achieved, it can be ticked off otherwise the remaining portion can be noted down. The following chart can be made for weekly schedule:

	Mathematics		*English*		*General Knowledge*	
	Target	*Done/ To do*	*Target*	*Done/ To do*	*Target*	*Done/ To do*
Monday						
Tuesday						
Wednesday						
Thursday						
Friday						
Saturday						
Sunday						

Peak Period: Every person has his/her own peak period i.e. the time when they have maximum concentration. For example, some students may have their peak period during early morning others may have it late night. Difficult chapters should be done during this time.

Class-School/College/Coaching	
Self Study	N U M B E R
Transportation	
Relaxation - TV, Net surfing etc.	O F
Physical Exercise	H O U R S
Daily routine (Brush, bath etc.)	
Sleep/Rest	

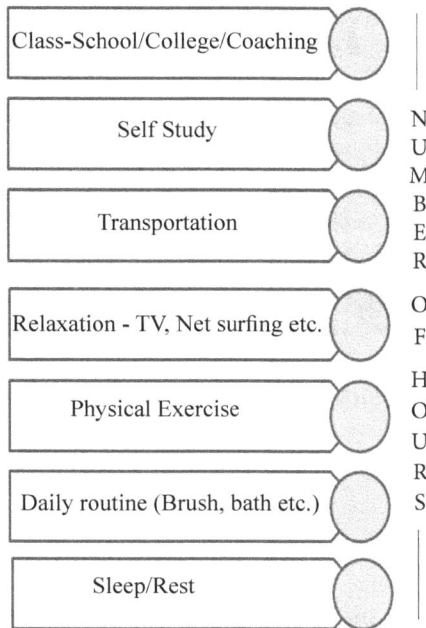

Self Reward : Some self rewards like watching a movie or a favourite TV programme can be awarded if the weekly schedule is accomplished.

10. **Solve mock test**

    After completing the syllabus the students should solve the past year papers, the sample papers as well as the practice test papers. Many coaching institutes offer test series. The students may join them to gain more confidence.

11. **Do physical exercise**

    This is a must for every person throughout the year. Physical exercise keeps a person healthy and improves blood circulation, oxygenates the body, boosts decision making skills, improves memory, increases attention span etc.

12. **Minimise stress**

    It is natural to be tensed, stressed and anxious before any examination. Physical exercise is one of the best stress busters. Apart from physical exercise, one can practice 'Pranayam' (breathing exercise) and meditation to reduce stress.

13. **Eat a balanced diet**

    A balanced diet is very important to keep the body as well as the brain healthy. The students should stop eating any junk food about two months prior to the examination. Some of the foods which increase brain power are whole grains, lentil, pomegranate juice, nuts, avocado, little quantity of dark chocolate etc. All these food release memory-enhancing chemicals and help to focus.

14. **Drink adequate water**

Water enhances mental function. The brain may get dehydrated in the absence of adequate water. Hence, the students should drink at least 8-10 glasses of water everyday.

15. **Have a good night's sleep**

Along with proper diet and adequate water, 7-8 hours of sleep is very important to be successful. Good sleep improves concentration, memory and grades. It lowers stress and anxiety.

① Arithmetic Formulae

NUMBER SYSTEM

Types of Numbers

a) **Natural Number**

Counting numbers starting from one are called natural numbers. It is represented by the symbol N. 1, 2, 3 ...

b) **Whole Number**

Natural numbers along with zero are called whole numbers. It is represented by the symbol W. 0, 1, 2, 3 ...

c) **Integer**

Natural numbers, zero along with negative numbers together form the integers. It is represented by the symbol Z.

... –3, –2, –1, 0, 1, 2, 3 ...

d) **Even Number**

A number which is divisible by two is called an even number.

2, 4, 6, 8 ...

e) **Odd Number**

A number which is not divisible by two is called an odd number.

1, 3, 5, 7 ...

f) **Prime Number**

A number which has only two factors one and itself is called a prime number. There are 25 prime numbers between 1 and 100. They are: 2, 3, 5, 7, 11, 13, 17, 19, 23, 29, 31, 37, 41, 43, 47, 53, 59, 61, 67, 71, 73, 79, 83, 89 and 97.

g) **Twin Prime**

A twin prime is a prime number that differs from another prime number by two. For example, 3 and 5, 5 and 7 ...

h) **Composite Number**

A number which has more than two factors is called a composite number. 4, 6, 8, 9, 10, 12, 14, 15, 16, 18 ...

i) **Co-prime Number**

Two numbers are said to be co-prime or relatively prime if their HCF is 1. For example, 2, 3 ; 3, 7 ...

Properties of prime and co-prime numbers

(i)   1 is neither prime nor composite.

(ii) 2 is the only even prime number.

(iii) Let p be a prime number. If p divides a^2, then p divides a, where a is a positive integer.

(iv) All prime numbers are co-prime to each other.

(v)   Any two consecutive integers are always co-prime.

(vi) Sum of any two co-prime numbers is always co-prime with their product.

(vii) 1 is co-prime with all numbers.

Fundamental Theorem of Arithmetic: Every composite number can be factorized as a product of primes. This factorization is unique apart from the order in which prime factors occur.

j)   **Rational Number**

A number which can be put in the form p/q where p and q are integers and $q \neq 0$ is called a rational number. It is represented by the symbol Q. For example, –3/5, 19, 2/9...

Properties of rational number

(i)   There are infinitely many rational numbers between any two given rational numbers.

(ii) If $x = p/q$ be a rational number, such that the prime factorisation of q is of the form $2^n 5^m$, where n, m are non-negative integers, then x has a decimal expansion which terminates.

(iii) If $x = p/q$ be a rational number, such that the prime factorisation of q is not of the form $2^n 5^m$, where n, m are non-negative integers, then x has a decimal expansion which is non-terminating repeating.

(iv) Rational numbers are either terminating or non-terminating recurring decimal.

k)   **Irrational Number**

A number which is neither terminating nor non-terminating repeating is known as an irrational number. For example, $\sqrt{2}$, $\sqrt{3}$, $\sqrt{5}$ ...

l)   **Real Number**

Rational numbers along with irrational numbers are known as real numbers. For example, 7/8, 23, $\sqrt{7}$ ... Every real number can be uniquely represented on a number line.

Note: If r is a rational number other than 0 and s is an irrational number, then $r + s$, $r - s$, $r \times s$ and $r \div s$ are irrational numbers.

Properties of real numbers

For any real numbers a, b and c,

(i) **Closure Property of Addition**
   Sum (or difference) of two real numbers equals a real number.

(ii) **Additive Identity**
   $a + 0 = a$

(iii) **Additive Inverse**
   $a + (-a) = 0$

(iv) **Associative Property of Addition**
   $(a + b) + c = a + (b + c)$

(v) **Commutative Property of Addition**
   $a + b = b + a$

(vi) **Definition of Subtraction**
   $a - b = a + (-b)$

(vii) **Closure Property of Multiplication**
   Product (or quotient if denominator $\neq 0$) of two real numbers equals a real number

(viii) **Multiplicative Identity**
   $a \times 1 = a$

(ix) **Multiplicative Inverse**
   $a \times (1/a) = 1 \ (a \neq 0)$

(x) **Multiplication by zero**
   $a \times 0 = 0$

(xi) **Commutative Property of Multiplication**
   $a \times b = b \times a$

(xii) **Associative Property of Multiplication**
   $(a \times b) \times c = a \times (b \times c)$

(xiii) **Distributive Law**
   $a(b + c) = ab + ac$

(xiv) **Definition of Division**
   $$\frac{a}{b} = a\left(\frac{1}{b}\right)$$

Even-Odd Relations

- Odd Integer $\times$ Odd Integer = Odd Integer
- Even Integer $\times$ Even Integer = Even Integer
- Odd Integer $\times$ Even Integer = Even Integer
- Odd Integer $+$ Odd Integer = Even Integer
- Odd Integer $-$ Odd Integer = Even Integer

$^{Odd} = Odd$

$^{Even} = Even$

$^{Odd} = Even$

Rules for Integer Operations

Addition (When signs are the same)

(i) Keep the sign.

(ii) Add.

Addition (When signs are different)

1. Keep the sign of the number that is farthest from zero.
2. Subtract the smaller number from the bigger number.

Subtraction

1. Change the subtraction sign to an addition sign.
2. Change the sign of the second number.
3. Follow addition rules.

Multiplication/Division

1. If there is an even number of negative signs, the answer will be positive.
2. If there is an odd number of negative signs, the answer will be negative.

BINARY NUMBER SYSTEM

Decimal Number System

The number system which uses ten digits- 0, 1, 2, 3, 4, 5, 6, 7, 8 and 9 is known as decimal number system.

Binary Number System

The number system which uses only two digits 0 and 1 is known as binary number system.

Note: Computers use binary digits commonly known as bit.

In computers,

1 Byte = 8 bits

1 Kilobyte = 1024 Byte

1 Megabyte = 1024 Kilobyte

1 Gigabyte = 1024 Megabyte

1 Terabyte = 1024 Gigabyte

Mathematics Formulae

Base of a Number System

The base of a number system is equal to the number of digits used in that system.

- The base of decimal system is 10.
- The base of binary system is 2.

Decimal to Binary Conversion

(i) Divide the number of the decimal system by 2.

(ii) Write the remainder as 0 if there is no remainder.

(iii) Divide the quotient by 2.

(iv) Continue the process till the quotient becomes 0 and the remainder is 1.

(v) Write the remainder from down upwards in left to right manner to get the binary number.

Binary to Decimal Conversion

1. Write the binary number.

2. Write 2^0, 2^1, 2^2, 2^3, 2^4, ... under each digit of the binary number starting from the right.

3. Cross out those powers of 2 which are under 0 of the binary number.

4. Add the remaining powers of 2.

Binary Addition

a) $0 + 0 = 0$

b) $0 + 1 = 1$

c) $1 + 0 = 1$

d) $1 + 1 = 0$ (carry 1)

Binary Subtraction

a) $0 - 0 = 0$

b) $1 - 0 = 1$

c) $1 - 1 = 0$

d) $10 - 1 = 1$

e) $0 - 1 =$ Borrow 1

Binary Multiplication

a) $0 \times 0 = 0$

b) $0 \times 1 = 0$

c) $1 \times 0 = 0$

d) $1 \times 1 = 1$

Binary Division

Binary division is similar to decimal long division.

Note: All fractions do not have an exact binary representation.

FACTORS AND MULTIPLES

Factor : A number is a factor of another number if the second number

Multiple : A number is a multiple of another number if it is divisible by the second number. For example, 6 is a multiple of 3.

Properties of Factors

(i) Every natural number is a factor of itself.

(ii) 1 is the factor of every number.

(iii) Every number is a factor of zero.

(iv) Every number other than 1 has at least two factors, namely the number itself and 1.

Properties of Multiples

(i) Every number is a multiple of 1.

(ii) Every number is a multiple of itself.

(iii) Zero (0) is a multiple of every number.

(iv) Every multiple except zero is either equal to or greater than any of its factors.

(v) The product of two or more factors is the multiple of each factor.

(vi)

Divisibility Rules

Divisible by	Rule
2	The last digit is even 0, 2, 4, 6, 8
3	The sum of the digits is divisible by 3
4	The last 2 digits are divisible by 4
5	The last digit is 0 or 5
6	The number is divisible by both 2 and 3
7	Double the last digit and subtract it from the rest of the number. If the answer is: 0, or divisible by 7 (The process may be repeated several times)
8	The last three digits are divisible by 8

9	The sum of the digits is divisible by 9
10	The number ends in 0
11	If the difference between the sum of the digits at odd places and the sum of the digits at even places is 0, or divisible by 11
12	The number is divisible by both 3 and 4

Euclid's Division Lemma

Given positive integers a and b, there exist unique integers q and r satisfying $a = bq + r$ $r < b$.

Note: A *lemma* is a proven statement used for proving another statement.

Euclid's Division Algorithm

The HCF of any two positive integers c and d, with $c > d$, is obtained as follows:

                           q and r where $c = dq + r$ and $r < d$.

2. If $r = 0$, the HCF is d. If   , apply Euclid's lemma to d and r.
3. Continue the process till the remainder is zero. The divisor at this stage will be HCF (c, d).
   Also, HCF(c, d) = HCF(d, r).

Note: An *algorithm*
procedure for solving a type of problem.

LCM and HCF

If a and b are positive integers then,

    LCM $(a, b) \times$ HCF $(a, b) = a \times b$

    If a, b, c are positive integers then,

    LCM $(a, b, c) \times$ HCF $(a, b, c$ $a \times b \times c$

    LCM $(a, b, c) = \dfrac{a.b.c \, \text{HCF}(a,b,c)}{\text{HCF}(a,b).\text{HCF}(b,c).\text{HCF}(a,c)}$

    HCF $(a, b, c) = \dfrac{a.b.c \, \text{LCM}(a,b,c)}{\text{LCM}(a,b).\text{LCM}(b,c).\text{LCM}(a,c)}$

FRACTION AND DECIMAL

Types of Fractions

Vulgar Fraction

A fraction consisting of an integer numerator and a non-zero denominator is called a common or a vulgar fraction.

For example, $\dfrac{9}{7}, \dfrac{3}{4}$

Proper Fraction

Fractions whose numerators are less than the denominators are called proper fractions.

For example, $\dfrac{3}{7}, \dfrac{8}{11}$

Improper Fraction

Fractions with the numerator either equal to or greater than the denominator are called improper fraction.

For example, $\dfrac{91}{23}, \dfrac{3}{2}$

Mixed Fraction

A combination of a proper fraction and a whole number is called a mixed fraction. For example, 21/3, 42/5

Properties of Fractions

(i)   Addition $\dfrac{a}{b} + \dfrac{c}{d} = \dfrac{ad + bc}{bd}$

(ii) Subtraction $\dfrac{a}{b} - \dfrac{c}{d} = \dfrac{ad - bc}{bd}$

(iii) Multiplication $\dfrac{a}{b} \times \dfrac{c}{d} = \dfrac{ac}{bd}$

(iv) Division $\dfrac{\frac{a}{b}}{\frac{c}{d}} = \dfrac{a}{b} \div \dfrac{c}{d} = \dfrac{a}{b} \times \dfrac{d}{c} = \dfrac{ad}{bc}$

(v)   The value of a fraction is not altered if both the numerator and denominator are multiplied or divided by the same number.

(vi) Reciprocal of a is $\dfrac{1}{a}$.

(vii) 1 and -1 are reciprocal of itself.

(viii) The reciprocal of zero does not exist.

Properties of Decimals

(i) A decimal fraction does not change if we add some zeros to the right of it. For example, 14.7 = 14.7000

(ii) A decimal fraction does not change if zeros are omitted from the end. For example, 0.00456000 = 0.00456

(iii) A decimal fraction will be increased by 10, 100, 1000,... times if the decimal point is shifted by one, two, three, ... places to the right respectively.

Mathematics Formulae

(iv) A decimal fraction will be decreased by 10, 100,1000,... times if the decimal point is shifted by one, two, three, ... places to the left respectively.

SQUARE AND SQUARE ROOT

If a natural number m can be expressed as n^2 i.e. $m = n \times n$, where n is also a natural number, then m is a **square number**. Square numbers are also called perfect squares.

Number	Square	Number	Square
1	1	11	121
2	4	12	144
3	9	13	169
4	16	14	196
5	25	15	225
6	36	16	256
7	49	17	289
8	64	18	324
9	81	19	361
10	100	20	400

Properties of Square Numbers

(i) All square numbers end with 0, 1, 4, 5, 6 or 9 at unit's place.

(ii) (a) If the last digit of a number is 1 or 9, its square ends in 1 and the number formed by its preceding digits must be divisible by four.

(b) If the last digit of a number is 2 or 8, its square ends in 4 and the preceding digit must be even.

(c) If the last digit of a number is 3 or 7, its square ends in 9 and the number formed by its preceding digits must be divisible by four.

(d) If the last digit of a number is 4 or 6, its square ends in 6 and the preceding digit must be odd.

(e) If the last digit of a number is 5, its square ends in 25.

(iii) A natural number having 2, 3, 7 or 8 at the one's place is never a perfect square.

(iv) A natural number with 0, 1, 4, 5, 6 or 9 at the one's place may or may not be a square number. Eg. 121 is a square number but 221 is not a square number.

(v)   The square of an even natural number is always even.

(vi) The square of an odd natural number is always odd.

(vii) The square of any odd number can be expressed as the sum of two consecutive positive integers.

(viii) Square numbers can only have even number of zeros at the end.

(ix) Factors of every square number can be grouped in pairs.

(x)   There are *2n* non perfect square numbers between any two consecutive square numbers *n* and *(n + 1)*.

(xi) A *n* digit natural number has either *2n* or *2n -1* digits in its square.

(xii) A perfect square leaves a remainder 0 or 1 when divided by 3.

(xiii) A perfect square can be expressed as a sum of successive odd natural numbers starting with 1.

(xiv) The square of any odd natural number can be expressed as the sum of two consecutive positive integers.

(xv) The square of a natural number greater than 1 can be written as

    (a) multiple of 3 or multiple of 3 plus 1.

    (b) multiple of 4 or multiple of 4 plus 1.

Square Root

Square root is the inverse operation of square. In other words, square root of a number a is a number y such that $y^2 = a$.

Properties of Square Root

(i)   Every non-negative real number a has a unique non-negative square root, called the principal root, which is denoted by $\sqrt{a}$.

(ii) Every positive number a has two square roots: $\sqrt{a}$, which is positive, and $-\sqrt{a}$, which is negative. Together, these two roots are denoted as $\pm \sqrt{a}$.

(iii) The square root of x is rational if and only if x is a rational number that can be represented as a ratio of two perfect squares.

$$\sqrt{x^2} = |x| = \begin{cases} x, & \text{if } x \geq 0 \\ -x, & \text{if } x < 0. \end{cases}$$

(iv) For all real numbers x

(v) $\sqrt{xy} = \sqrt{x}\sqrt{y}$ For all non-negative real numbers x and y,

$$\sqrt{\frac{x}{y}} = \frac{\sqrt{x}}{\sqrt{y}} \text{ where } x > 0, y > 0$$

(vi) If a perfect square is of n digits, then its square root has $\frac{n}{2}$ digits if n is even and $\frac{(n+1)}{2}$ if n is odd.

CUBE AND CUBE ROOT

Numbers obtained when a number is multiplied by itself three times are known as cube numbers. In other words, a natural number n is a perfect cube, if there exists a natural number m such that:
$n = m \times m \times m = m^3$

Number	Cube	Number	Cube
1	1	11	1331
2	8	12	1728
3	27	13	2197
4	64	14	2744
5	125	15	3375
6	216	16	4096
7	343	17	4913
8	512	18	5832
9	729	19	6859
10	1000	20	8000

Properties of Cube

(i) A perfect cube can be expressed as a product of triplets of equal factors.

(ii) There are ten perfect cubes from 1 to 1000.

(iii) Cubes of all even natural numbers are even.

(iv) Cubes of all odd natural numbers are odd.

(v) Cubes of negative integers are negative.

(vi) The product of the cubes of two numbers is equal to the cube of their products. For any two natural numbers a and b,
$$a^3 \times b^3 = (a \times b)^3.$$

(vii) The cube of a rational number is the cube of its numerator divided by the cube of its denominator.
$$\left(\frac{p}{q} \right)^3 = \frac{p^3}{q^3}$$

(viii) Numbers like 1729, 4104, 13832, are known as Hardy–Ramanujan Numbers. They can be expressed as sum of two cubes in two different ways. For example,
$$1729 = 1728 + 1 = 12^3 + 1^3$$
$$1729 = 1000 + 729 = 10^3 + 9^3$$

Cube Root

Cube root is the inverse operation of cube. In other words, cube root of a number a is a number y such that $y^3 = a$.

Properties of Cube Root

For all non-negative real numbers a and b,

(i) $\sqrt[3]{a+b} \neq \sqrt[3]{a} + \sqrt[3]{b}$

(ii) $\sqrt[3]{a-b} \neq \sqrt[3]{a} - \sqrt[3]{b}$

(iii) $\sqrt[3]{a \times b} = \sqrt[3]{a} \times \sqrt[3]{b}$

(iv) $\sqrt[3]{\dfrac{a}{b}} = \dfrac{\sqrt[3]{a}}{\sqrt[3]{b}}$

MATHEMATICAL OPERATION

The rule for simplifying mathematical expressions involving multiple operations is BODMAS. BODMAS stands for the order of operation.

B	Bracket
O	Order (Power, Square Root etc)
D	Division
M	Multiplication
A	Addition
S	Subtraction

Bracket Rules

If the mathematical expression contains more than one bracket, then the order of solving the bracket is:

(i) First bracket to be removed is the line bracket or bar bracket or

(ii) Second bracket to be removed is the common bracket ( ).

(iii) Third bracket to be removed is the curly bracket { }.

(iv) Fourth bracket to be removed is the square bracket [ ] .

Modulus of a Real Number

Modulus of a real number a

$$|a| = \begin{cases} a & if\ a \geq 0 \\ -a & if\ a < 0 \end{cases}$$

PERCENTAGE

A percentage is a fraction whose denominator is 100.

Percentage change

$$\% \text{ Change} = \frac{\text{New Value} - \text{Original Value}}{\text{Original Value}} \times 100$$

Percentage Error

$$\% \text{ Error} = \frac{\text{Error}}{\text{Real Value}} \times 100$$

Original value

$$\text{Original Value} = \frac{\text{New Value}}{100 + \% \text{Change}} \times 100$$

Percentage increase

$$\text{New Value} = \frac{100 + \text{Percentage Increase}}{100} \times \text{Original Value}$$

Percentage decrease

$$\text{New Value} = \frac{100 - \text{Percentage Decrease}}{100} \times \text{Original Value}$$

Relation Between Fraction, Decimal and Percent

Fraction	Decimal	Percent	Fraction	Decimal	Percent
$\frac{1}{2}$	0.5	50%	$\frac{3}{5}$	0.6	60%
$\frac{2}{2}$	1.0	100%	$\frac{4}{5}$	0.8	80%
$\frac{1}{3}$	$0.\bar{3}$	$33\frac{1}{3}\%$	$\frac{5}{5}$	1.0	100%
$\frac{2}{3}$	$0.\bar{6}$	$66\frac{2}{3}\%$	$\frac{1}{8}$	0.125	12.5%
$\frac{3}{3}$	1.0	100%	$\frac{2}{8}$	0.25	25%
$\frac{1}{4}$	0.25	25%	$\frac{3}{8}$	0.375	37.5%
$\frac{2}{4}$	0.5	50%	$\frac{4}{8}$	0.5	50%

$\dfrac{3}{4}$	0.75	75%	$\dfrac{5}{8}$	0.625	62.5%
$\dfrac{4}{4}$	1.0	100%	$\dfrac{6}{8}$	0.75	75%
$\dfrac{1}{5}$	0.2	20%	$\dfrac{7}{8}$	0.875	87.5%
$\dfrac{2}{5}$	0.4	40%	$\dfrac{8}{8}$	1.0	100%

Conversion of Fraction or Decimal into Percentage and Vice Versa

To convert a fraction or decimal into percentage, multiply it by 100.

For example, $\dfrac{4}{5} \times 100 = 80\%$

To convert a percentage into fraction or decimal, divide it by 100.

For example, 38.9 % is same as $38.9 \div 100 = 0.389$

PROFIT AND LOSS

Cost Price : The price, at which an article is purchased, is called its cost price, *C.P.*

Selling Price : The price, at which an article is sold, is called its selling price, *S.P.*

If S.P. is greater than C.P., the seller is said to have

Loss : If S.P. is less than C.P., the seller is said to have incurred a loss.

Key Terms and Formulae

(i) Gain = (S.P.) - (C.P.)

(ii) Loss = (C.P.) - (S.P.)

(iii)Loss or gain is always calculated on C.P.

(iv) Gain Percentage: (Gain%)

$$\text{Gain}\% = \left(\frac{\text{Gain} \times 100}{\text{C.P.}} \right)$$

(v) Loss Percentage: (Loss%)

$$\text{Loss}\% = \left(\frac{\text{Loss} \times 100}{\text{C.P.}} \right)$$

Mathematics Formulae

(vi) Selling Price: (S.P.)

$$SP = \left[\frac{(100 + \text{Gain}\%)}{100} \times \text{C.P.} \right]$$

(vii) Selling Price: (S.P.)

$$SP = \left[\frac{(100 - \text{Loss}\%)}{100} \times \text{C.P.} \right]$$

(viii) Cost Price: (C.P.)

$$\text{C.P.} = \left[\frac{100}{(100 + \text{Gain}\%)} \times SP \right]$$

(ix) Cost Price: (C.P.)

$$\text{C.P.} = \left[\frac{100}{(100 - \text{Loss}\%)} \times \text{S.P.} \right]$$

(x) If a trader professes to sell his goods at cost price, but uses false weights, then

$$\text{Gain}\% = \left[\frac{\text{Error}}{(\text{True Value}) - (\text{Error})} \times 100 \right]\%$$

SALES TAX AND DISCOUNT

Marked Price

The printed price of an article is called its marked price or list price (MP).

Discount

Discount is a reduction given on marked price.

Discount = Marked Price – Sale Price.

Discount can be calculated when discount percentage is given.

Discount = Discount % of Marked Price

$$\text{Discount}\% = \frac{\text{Discount}}{\text{MP}} \times 100$$

where MP is the marked price.

Net Selling Price

The difference between the marked price and the discount is called the net selling price (SP).

SP = Marked Price – Discount

Banker's Discount

Banker's Discount is the difference between the value shown on a bond, share etc that is bought by a bank from a customer, and the amount that the customer actually receives from the bank. The banker's discount is kept by the bank as a payment. Thus, Banker's Discount is the simple interest on the face value for the period from the date on which the bill was discounted and the legally due date.

Bill of Exchange
A written order by one party (the drawer) to another (the drawee) to pay a certain sum either immediately (a sight bill) or on a fixed date (a term bill) for payment of goods or services received. The drawee accepts the bill by signing it.

Nominally Due Date
The exact date to which the bill of exchange is due for payment is known as nominally due date.

Legally Due Date
Three days (grace days) after the nominally due date is known as legally due date.

Note: When the date of the bill is not given, grace days are not to be added.

Key Terms and Formulae
(i) Banker's Discount = Simple Interest on the face value of the bill for unexpired time

$$= \frac{\text{Face Value} \times \text{Rate} \times \text{Time}}{100}$$

(ii) Banker's Gain = Banker's Discount – True Discount (for unexpired time)

$$= \text{Simple interest on True Discount}$$

$$= \frac{(\text{True Discount})^2}{\text{Present Worth}}$$

(iii) True Discount $= \sqrt{\text{Present Worth} \times \text{Banker's Gain}}$

(iv) True Discount = Simple Interest on the present worth for unexpired time

$$= \frac{\text{Present Worth} \times \text{Time} \times \text{Rate}}{100}$$

$$= \frac{\text{Face Value} \times \text{Rate} \times \text{Time}}{100 + (\text{Rate} \times \text{Time})}$$

(v) Face Value $= \dfrac{\text{Banker's Discount} \times \text{True Discount}}{\text{Banker's Discount} - \text{True Discount}}$

(vi) Present Worth = Face Value − True Discount

(vii) True Discount = $\dfrac{\text{Banker's Gain} \times 100}{\text{Rate} \times \text{Time}}$

(viii) Present Worth = $\dfrac{\text{Face Value}}{1 + \text{Time}\left(\dfrac{\text{Rate}}{100}\right)}$

Sales Tax

Sales tax is charged on the sale of an item by the government and is

Added Tax) rate for various categories of items.

Sales tax = Tax% of Bill Amount

Note: If both discount and sales tax are given in a problem, then the

ALLIGATION AND MIXTURE

Alligation

ingredients at the given price must be mixed to produce a mixture of desired price.

Mean Price

The cost of a unit quantity of the mixture is called the mean price.

Rule of Alligation

If two ingredients are mixed, then

$$\left(\frac{\text{Quantity of cheaper}}{\text{Quantity of dearer}}\right) = \left(\frac{\text{C.P. of dearer} - \text{Mean Price}}{\text{Mean price} - \text{C.P. of cheaper}}\right)$$

It can be represented as:

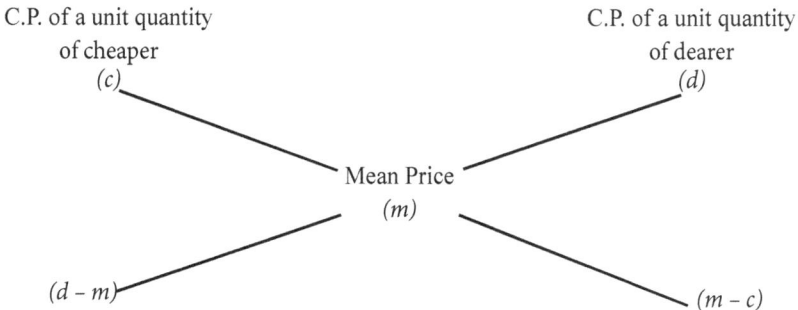

C.P. of a unit quantity
of cheaper
(c)

C.P. of a unit quantity
of dearer
(d)

Mean Price
(m)

(d − m)

(m − c)

Hence,(Cheaper quantity) : (Dearer quantity) = $(d - m) : (m - c)$.

Suppose, a container contains x units of liquid from which y units are taken out and replaced by water.

After n operations the quantity of pure liquid

$$= \left[x \left(1 - \frac{y}{x} \right)^n \right] \text{units}.$$

Mixture of More Than Two Elements

(i) If n different vessels of equal size are filled with the mixture of P and Q in the ratio $p_1 : q_1, p_2 : q_2, ..., p_n : q_n$ and content of all these vessels are mixed in one large vessel, then

$$\frac{\text{Quantity of P}}{\text{Quantity of Q}} = \frac{\dfrac{p_1}{p_1+q_1} + \dfrac{p_2}{p_2+q_2} + ... + \dfrac{p_n}{p_n+q_n}}{\dfrac{q_1}{p_1+q_1} + \dfrac{q_2}{p_2+q_2} + ... + \dfrac{q_n}{p_n+q_n}}$$

(ii) If n different vessels of sizes $x_1, x_2, ..., x_n$ are filled with the mixture of P and Q in the ratio $p_1 : q_1, p_2 : q_2, ..., p_n : q_n$ and content of all these vessels are mixed in one large vessel, then

$$\frac{\text{Quantity of P}}{\text{Quantity of Q}} = \frac{\dfrac{p_1 x_1}{p_1+q_1} + \dfrac{p_2 x_2}{p_2+q_2} + ... + \dfrac{p_n x_n}{p_n+q_n}}{\dfrac{q_1 x_1}{p_1+q_1} + \dfrac{q_2 x_2}{p_2+q_2} + ... + \dfrac{q_n x_n}{p_n+q_n}}$$

(iii) If a vessel contains 'x' litres of liquid A and if 'y' litres be withdrawn and replaced by liquid B, and the operation is repeated 'n' times in all, then :

$$\frac{\text{Quantity of liquid A after } n^{\text{th}} \text{ operation}}{\text{Initial quantity of liquid of A}} = \left[\frac{x-y}{x} \right]^n = \left[1 - \frac{y}{x} \right]^n$$

(iv) p gram of an ingredient solution has $a\%$ ingredient in it. To increase the ingredient content to $b\%$ in the solution

$$\text{Quantity of ingredient need to be added} = \frac{p(b-a)}{100-b}$$

INTEREST

Principal : The money borrowed is known as principal.

Rate : The percentage of a sum of money which is charged or paid for the use of money is known as rate of interest.

Interest : The extra money which is paid for using the principal is known as interest.

$$\text{Simple Interest} = \frac{\text{Principal} \times \text{Rate} \times \text{Time}}{100}$$

Amount = Principal + Simple Interest

Compound Interest : The interest earned on capital when the interest is periodically added to the principal.

If P = Principal, R = Rate, T = Time

When Compound Interest reckoned

(i) **Annually**

$$\text{Amount} = P\left\{1 + \frac{R}{100}\right\}^{T}$$

(ii) **Half-Yearly**

$$\text{Amount} = P\left\{1 + \frac{R}{2 \times 100}\right\}^{2 \times T}$$

i.e. Rate = R/2 and Time = $2 \times T$

(iii) **Quarterly**

$$\text{Amount} = P\left\{1 + \frac{R}{4 \times 100}\right\}^{4 \times T}$$

i.e. Rate = R/4 and Time = $4 \times T$

(iv) If Principal = P, Rate = r_1 % for 1st year, r_2 % for 2nd year, r_3 % for 3rd year and so on and in the last r_n % for nth year

$$\text{Amount} = P\left\{\left(1 + \frac{r_1}{100}\right)\left(1 + \frac{r_2}{100}\right)\left(1 + \frac{r_3}{100}\right)\ldots\left(1 + \frac{r_n}{100}\right)\right\}$$

(v) If Principal = P, Rate = R and Time = $a\dfrac{b}{c}$ *i.e.* Time is in fraction.

$$\text{Amount} = P \left(1 + \frac{R}{100}\right)^a \left(1 + \frac{R}{100} \times \frac{b}{c}\right)$$

(vi) Compound Interest = $P\left[\left(1 + \dfrac{R}{100}\right)^T - 1\right]$

RATIO AND PROPORTION

Ratio

A ratio is a comparison between two numbers or between two quantities with the same units. For example, the ratio of two numbers a and b is the fraction $-$, usually expressed in the lowest term. The

Equivalent Ratio

Two ratios can be compared by converting them to like fractions. If the two fractions are equal, the two given ratios are equivalent.

Proportion

A proportion is an equation which states that two ratios are equal i.e. *a:b :: c:d*. The order of the terms is important in proportion.

In a proportion, the outermost terms are known as *extremes* and the inner two terms are known as *means*.

Also, the product of extremes = the product of means

Or, *ad = bc.*

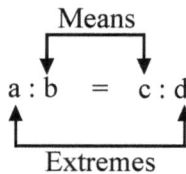

TIME AND WORK

Work from Days

If A can do a piece of work in n days, then A's 1 day's work is $\dfrac{1}{n}$.

Days from Work

If A's 1 day's work is $-$ n days.

Ratio of Work Done

If A is twice as good a workman as B, then:

Ratio of work done by A and B = 2 : 1

Ratio of time taken by A and B to finish a work = 1 : 2

Key Terms and Formulae

(i) If A can do a piece of work in a days and B can do the same piece of work in b days by working alone, then A and B together can finish the work in $\dfrac{ab}{a+b}$ days

(ii) If A, B and C can complete a piece of work in a, b and c days respectively by working alone, then they will together complete the work in $\dfrac{abc}{ab+bc+ca}$ days

(iii) If A and B working together can finish a piece of work in p days, A working alone can finish in q days, then B working alone will finish the work in $\dfrac{pq}{q-p}$ days

(iv) A and B working together can finish a piece of work in p days, B and C working together can finish a piece of work in q days and C and A working together can finish a piece of work in r days then

    a) A, B and C working together can finish the work in $\dfrac{2pqr}{pq+qr+rp}$ days

    b) A alone can finish the work in $\dfrac{2pqr}{pq+qr-rp}$ days

    c) B alone can finish the work in $\dfrac{2pqr}{qr+rp-pq}$ days

(v) If A working alone takes a days more than A and B working together, B working alone takes b days more than A and B working together then the time taken by A and B to complete the work is equal to:

    $\sqrt{ab}$ days

(vi) If a men and b women can complete a piece of work in n days then c men and d women will complete the same work in $\dfrac{nab}{bc+ad}$ days

(vii) Let two groups of people have the same efficiency. If M_1 men can do W_1 work in D_1 days working H_1 hours per day and if M_2 men can do W_2 work in D_2 days working H_2 hours per day, then:

$$\frac{M_1 D_1 H_1}{W_1} = \frac{M_2 D_2 H_2}{W_2}$$

PIPES AND CISTERNS

Inlet :
it, is known as an inlet.

Outlet : A pipe connected with a reservoir or a tank or a cistern that empties it, is known as an outlet.

Filling and Emptying of Pipe

(i) If a x $\dfrac{1}{x}$.

(ii) If a pipe can empty a tank in y hours, then the part emptied in 1 hour $= \dfrac{1}{y}$.

x hours and another pipe can empty the full tank in y hours (where $y > x$), then on opening both the pipes the part emptied in 1 hour $= \dfrac{1}{y} - \dfrac{1}{x}$

x hours and another pipe can empty the full tank in y hours (where $y > x$), then on opening both the pipes $= \dfrac{1}{x} - \dfrac{1}{y}$

(v) If x y is the time taken to

container $= \dfrac{xy}{y-x}$

(vi) Let x y be the

container $= \dfrac{xy}{x+y}$

(vii) Let there be three inlet pipes X, Y and Z. Let x, y, and z be the

working alone. If all the three pipes are opened together, then

$$= \dfrac{xyz}{xy + yz + zx}$$

(viii) Let there be two inlet pipes X and Y and one outlet pipe Z. If x

container when all the pipes are open, then time taken to empty the container

$$= \dfrac{xyz}{xz + yz - xy}$$

(ix) If d_1, d_2 and d_3
where $d_1 > d_2 > d_3$
when all the pipes are open is given by

$$\text{Time required} = \left[\frac{(\text{Time taken by largest pipe}) \times d_1^2}{d_1^2 + d_2^2 + d_3^2} \right]$$

(x) If an inlet pipe X is k times faster and takes x minutes less time than inlet pipe Y then

together is given by $= \dfrac{kx}{(k-1)^2}$

$$= \frac{x}{k-1}$$
$$\frac{kx}{k-1}$$

CLOCKS AND CALENDAR

Minute Space
For calculation purpose, the dial of a clock is taken as a circle whose circumference is divided into 60 equal parts, known as minute space.

Hour Hand and Minute Hand
A clock has two hands. The smaller hand is called the hour hand while the larger one is called the minute hand.

Properties of a Clock
(i) There are 360 degrees of angular measurement in a circle. This is applied to the clock problem because a standard non-digital clock is generally a circle.

(ii) The angle between two consecutive hours is 30 degrees.

(iii) The angle between two consecutive minutes is 6 degrees.

(vi) In every hour, both the hands coincide once.

(v) The hands are in the same straight line when they are coincident or opposite to each other.

(vi) When the two hands are at right angles, they are 15 minute spaces apart.

(vii) Angle traced by hour hand in 12 hours = 360°

(viii) Angle traced by minute hand in 60 minutes = 360°

(ix) If a clock shows 7.20, when the correct time is 7, it is said to be 20 minutes too fast.

x) On the other hand, if it indicates 7.40, when the correct time is 8, it is said to be 20 minutes too slow.

Properties of a Calendar

(i)   1 week = 7 days

(ii)   1 month = 30 or 31 days (except February, for calculation purpose 30 is taken unless the name of the month is mentioned).

(iii) A period of ten years is known as a decade.

(iv)   A period of 100 years is known as a century.

(v)   The first day of a century is either Monday, Tuesday, Thursday or Saturday.

(vi)   The last day of a century cannot be Tuesday, Thursday or Saturday.

(vii) An ordinary year has 365 days (February = 28 days)

(viii) A leap year has 366 days (February = 29 days)

(ix)   A leap year comes once in four years.

(x)   The year which is divisible by four is a leap year, if it is not a century. For a century to be a leap year it should be divisible by 400.

(xi)   Every 4th century is a leap year and no other century is a leap year. For example, 2000 is a leap year but 2100 is not a leap year.

(xii) There are 52 weeks in a year.

Odd Days

The number of days more than the complete weeks are called odd days.

1 Ordinary year	=	52 Weeks + 1 odd day
1 Leap year	=	52 Weeks + 2 odd days
1 Century	=	76 Ordinary years + 24 Leap years
	=	76 Odd days + 48 Odd days
	=	124 Odd days
	=	17 weeks + 5 odd days

Number of odd days	0	1	2	3	4	5	6
Day of the week	Sunday	Monday	Tuesday	Wednesday	Thursday	Friday	Saturday

Working Rule When No Reference Day is Given

To find the day of the week on a particular date when no reference day is given

(i) Count the total number of odd days on the given date.

(ii) Use the above table to find out the day of the week.

Working Rule when Reference Day is Given

is given

(i) Count the total number of odd days for the period between the given date and the reference date. (Include the given date but exclude the reference date during counting).

(ii) The day of the week on the particular date is equal to the total number of odd days behind the reference date if the given date was behind the reference date and ahead of the reference date if the reference date was ahead of it.

SPEED, DISTANCE AND TIME

Key Terms and Formulae

$$\text{Distance} = \text{Speed} \times \text{Time}$$

$$\text{Speed} = \frac{\text{Distance}}{\text{Time}}$$

(i) In a race if P is n times as fast as Q and Q starts x metres ahead of P, then length of the race course so that both P and Q reach the

$$x\left(\frac{n}{n+1}\right) \text{meters}$$

(ii) If P can run p metres race in t_1 seconds and Q in t_2 seconds where $t_1 < t_2$ then P beats Q by a distance $= \dfrac{p}{t_2} \times (t_2 - t_1)$

(iii) If P covers a distance d_1 km at s_1 km/h and then d_2 km at s_2 km/h, then the average speed during the whole journey is

$$\frac{s_1 s_2 (d_1 + d_2)}{s_1 d_2 + s_2 d_1} km/h$$

(iv) If P goes from A to B at s_1 km/h and returns from B to A at s_2 km/h, then the average speed during the whole journey is

$$\frac{2 s_1 s_2}{s_1 + s_2} km/h$$

(v) If a man covers a certain distance at x km/h and an equal distance at y km/h and z km/h, then the average speed during the whole journey is $= \dfrac{3xyz}{(xy + yz + zx)} km/h$

(vi) If a body travels distance d_1, d_2, ... in time t_1, t_2, ... respectively then

$$\text{Average Speed} = \frac{\text{Total distance}}{\text{Total time}}$$

(vii) If the new speed of a body is a/b times the original speed then the change in time to cover the same distance is $\left(\frac{b}{a} - 1\right) \times$ original time.

(viii) If a body moves with speed s_1 km/h and covers a distance d km in time t_1 and then moves with speed s_2 km/h and covers the same distance in time t_2 then

$$\frac{\text{Product of speed}}{d} = \frac{s_1}{t_1} = \frac{s_2}{t_2} = \frac{\text{Difference of speed}}{\text{Difference of time}}$$

(ix) If the speed of the boat be x km/h and the speed of the stream be y km/h, then

    a) The speed of the boat upstream (direction opposite to the stream) = $(x - y)$km/h

    b) The speed of the boat downstream (direction along the stream) = $(x + y)$km/h

    c) Speed of the stream = $\frac{1}{2}$ (Down stream speed − upstream speed)

TRAIN PROBLEMS

(i) Time taken by a train of length l metres to pass a pole or a signal post or a standing man is equal to the time taken by the train to cover l metres.

(ii) Time taken by a train of length l metres to pass a stationery object of length p metres is the time taken by the train to cover $(l + p)$ metres.

(iii) Suppose two trains or two bodies are moving in the same direction at u m/s and v m/s, where $u > v$, then their relative speed is equal to $(u - v)$ m/s.

(iv) Suppose two trains or two bodies are moving in opposite directions at u m/s and v m/s, then their relative speed is equal to $(u + v)$ m/s.

(v) If two trains of length a metres and b metres are moving in opposite directions at u m/s and v m/s, then the time taken by the trains to cross each other is $\frac{(a+b)}{u+v}$ sec

(vi) If two trains of length a metres and b metres are moving in the same directions at u m/s and v m/s, then the time taken by the faster train to cross the slower train is $\frac{(a+b)}{u-v}$ sec

(vii) If two trains (or bodies) start at the same time from points A and B towards each other and after crossing they take a and b sec in reaching B and A respectively, then:

$$(\text{A's speed}) : (\text{B's speed}) = (\sqrt{b} : \sqrt{a})$$

SEQUENCE AND PROGRESSION

Sequence

is known as a sequence.

Or

A function whose domain is the set of natural numbers or some subset of it of the type {1, 2, 3...k} is known as a sequence.

Finite Sequence

Infinite Sequence

sequence.

Fibonacci Sequence

The sequence 1, 1, 2, 3, 5, 8, ... is known as Fibonacci Sequence. It is described by the following rule:

$a_1 = a_2 = 1$

$a_3 = a_1 + a_2$

$a_n = a_{n-2} + a_{n-1}, n > 2$

Progression

Arithmetic Progression (A.P)

An arithmetic progression (A.P.) is a sequence in which terms increase or decrease regularly by the same constant. This constant is called common difference (d) of the A.P.

Standard Form of A.P

If 'a' 'd' is the common difference, then the standard form of A.P is given by

$$a, (a+d), (a+2d), (a+3d), (a+4d), ...$$

Consecutive Terms

For solving problems,

Three consecutive terms of an A.P are taken as

$$(a - d), a, (a + d).$$

Five consecutive terms of an A.P are taken as

$$(a - 2d), (a - d), a, (a + d), (a + 2d).$$

General Term

The nth term of the A.P. $= a_n = a + (n-1)d$. The nth term is also called the general term of A.P.

Sum of n Terms

The sum of n terms of the A.P. is

(i) $S_n = \dfrac{n}{2}\left[2a + (n-1)d\right]$

   where a is the first term and d is the common difference.

(ii) $S_n = \dfrac{n}{2}(a + a_n)$

   where a is the first term and a_n is the nth term of the A.P .

(iii) $S_n = \dfrac{n}{2}(a + l)$

   where a is the first term and l is the last term of the A.P.

Note:

- The common difference d of an A.P can be negative, positive or zero.
- A.P can be finite or infinite.
- An infinite A.P does not have any last term.

Properties of an A.P

(i) If a constant is added or subtracted to/from each term of an A.P., the resulting sequence is also an A.P.

(ii) If each term of an A.P. is multiplied by a constant, then the resulting sequence is also an A.P.

(iii) If each term of an A.P. is divided by a non-zero constant, then the resulting sequence is also an A.P.

(iv) Three numbers a, b, c are in A.P. if $2b = a + c$

Geometric Progression (G.P)

Definition

A sequence $a_1, a_2, a_3, ..., a_n$ is called geometric progression, if each term is non-zero and $\dfrac{a_{k+1}}{a_k} = r$ (constant), for $k \geq 1$

Mathematics Formulae

Standard Form of G.P

If 'a' is the first term and 'r' is the common ratio, then the standard form of G.P is given by a, ar, ar^2, ar^3, ...

Consecutive Terms

For solving problems,

Three consecutive terms of a G.P are taken as $\dfrac{a}{r}$, a, ar.

Five consecutive terms of a G.P are taken as $\dfrac{a}{r^2}$, $\dfrac{a}{r}$, a, ar, ar^2

General Term

The nth term of the G.P. is $a_n = ar^{n-1}$

where a is the first term and r is the common ratio.

Sum of n Terms

(i) If $r = 1$, the sum of n terms is given by, $S_n = na$

(ii) If $r \neq 1$, the sum of n terms of the G.P. is $S_n = a\left(\dfrac{1-r^n}{1-r}\right)$

Or,

$$S_n = a\left(\dfrac{r^n - 1}{r-1}\right)$$

where a is the first term, r is the common ratio.

Sum of Infinite Terms

The sum of infinite number of terms of the G.P is

$$S_\infty = \sum_{n=1}^{\infty} ar^{n-1} = \dfrac{a}{1-r} \text{ , where } -1 < r < 1$$

Properties of geometric progression

(i) If the common ratio is:
- Negative, the terms will alternate between positive and negative.
- Positive, the terms will all be the same sign as the initial term.
- Equal to 1, the progression is a constant sequence.
- Greater than 1, there will be exponential growth towards positive or negative infinity (depending on the sign of the initial term).
- Between -1 and 1 but not zero, there will be exponential decay towards zero.
- -1, the progression is an alternating sequence

(ii) Three numbers a, b, c are in G.P. if $b^2 = ac$.

Harmonic Progression (H.P)

The sequence a_1, a_2, a_3 ... are said to be in Harmonic Progression if their reciprocals $\dfrac{1}{a_1}, \dfrac{1}{a_2}, \dfrac{1}{a_3}...$ are in Arithmetic Progression.

Arithmetic, Geometric and Harmonic Mean

Arithmetic Mean

(i) If a,b,c (positive numbers) are in A.P, then b is called the arithmetic mean of a and c. It is given by $b = \dfrac{a+c}{2}$

(ii) The Arithmetic Mean of $x_1, x_2, ..., x_n$ is given by

$$\text{Arithmetic Mean} = \frac{1}{n}\sum_{i=1}^{n} x_i$$

Geometric Mean

(i) The Geometric Mean of two positive numbers a and b is given by

$$\text{Geometric Mean} = \sqrt{ab}$$

(ii) The Geometric Mean of $x_1, x_2, ..., x_n$ is given by

$$G = \sqrt[n]{x_1 x_2 \cdots x_n}$$

and hence

$$\log G = \frac{1}{n}\sum_{i=1}^{n} \log x_i$$

Or, the logarithm of the geometric mean is the arithmetic mean of the logarithm of numbers.

Harmonic Mean

(i) The Harmonic Mean of two positive numbers a and b is given by

$$\text{Harmonic Mean} = \frac{2ab}{a+b}$$

(ii) The Harmonic Mean H of the positive numbers $x_1, x_2, ..., x_n$ is defined to be the reciprocal of the arithmetic mean of the reciprocals of $x_1, x_2, ..., x_n$:

$$H = \left(\frac{1}{n}\cdot\sum_{i=1}^{n} x_i^{-1}\right)^{-1} = \frac{1}{\dfrac{1}{n}\cdot\left(\dfrac{1}{x_1}+\dfrac{1}{x_2}+\cdots+\dfrac{1}{x_n}\right)} = \frac{n}{\dfrac{1}{x_1}+\dfrac{1}{x_2}+\cdots+\dfrac{1}{x_n}}$$

Relationship between Various Mean

Arithmetic Mean and Geometric Mean

If a and b are two positive numbers then,

$$\text{Arithmetic Mean} - \text{Geometric Mean} = \frac{\left(\sqrt{a}-\sqrt{b}\right)^2}{2} \geq 0$$

Or Arithmetic Mean $\geq$ Geometric Mean

Arithmetic, Geometric and Harmonic Mean

For positive numbers,

(i) (Geometric Mean)^2 = Arithmetic Mean $\times$ Harmonic Mean

(ii) Arithmetic Mean > Geometric Mean > Harmonic Mean

Mathematics Formulae

PARTNERSHIP

Partnership

When two or more than two persons run a business jointly, they are called partners and the deal is known as partnership.

Simple Partnership

The partnership in which the capital of each partner is invested in the business for the same time period is known as simple partnership.

Compound Partnership

The partnership in which the capital of each partner is invested in the business for different time period is known as compound partnership.

Working and Sleeping Partners

A partner who manages the business is known as a working partner and the partner who simply invests the money is a sleeping partner.

Ratio of Divisions of Gains

(i) When investments of all the partners are for the same time, the gain or loss is distributed among the partners in the ratio of their investments.

Suppose A and B invest Rs. x and Rs. y respectively for the same time

P then
$$\frac{x \times P}{x + y}$$
$$\frac{y \times P}{x + y}$$

(ii) When investments are for different time periods, equivalent capitals are calculated for a unit of time by taking

(capital × number of units of time). Now gain or loss is divided in the ratio of these capitals.

Suppose A invests Rs. x for p years and B invests Rs. y for q years, then
$$\frac{\text{A's share of profit}}{\text{B's share of profit}} = \frac{xp}{yq}$$

(iii) If three partners A, B and C invest capitals Rs. x, Rs. y and Rs. z for a time period of a, b and c years respectively and if P is the
$$\text{Share of A} = \frac{axP}{ax + by + cz}$$
$$\text{Share of B} = \frac{byP}{ax + by + cz}$$

$$\text{Share of C} = \frac{czP}{ax + by + cz}$$

Ratio of Investment Period

If three partners A, B and C invest their capitals in the ratio of $x : y : z$ and gain is in the ratio of $p : q : r$ then,

$$\text{Ratio of time of Investment of A, B, C} = \frac{p}{x} : \frac{q}{y} : \frac{r}{z}$$

Ratio of Capital

If three partners A, B and C shared profit in the ratio of $p : q : r$ when the capital is invested for a time period of $a : b : c$ then,

$$\text{Ratio of invested capital of A, B, C} = \frac{p}{a} : \frac{q}{b} : \frac{r}{c}$$

STOCKS AND SHARES

Stock Capital

The total amount of money needed to run the company is called the stock capital.

Shares or Stock

The whole capital is divided into small units, called shares or stock.

showing the value of each share and the number of shares held by a person.

The person who subscribes in shares or stock is called a share holder or stock holder.

Dividend

Dividend is paid annually as per share or as a percentage.

Face Value

its Face Value or Nominal Value or Par Value.

Market Value

The stock of different companies are sold and bought in the open market through brokers at stock-exchanges. A share or stock is said to be:

(i) At premium or above par, if its market value is more than its face value.

(ii) At par, if its market value is the same as its face value.

(iii) At discount or below par, if its market value is less than its face value.

Thus, if a Rs. 100 stock is quoted at premium of 15, then market value of the stock = Rs.(100 + 15) = Rs. 115

Likewise, if a Rs. 100 stock is quoted at a discount of 6, then market value of the stock = Rs. (100 - 6) = Rs. 94

Brokerage

The broker's charge is called brokerage.

(i) When stock is purchased, brokerage is added to the cost price.

(ii) When stock is sold, brokerage is subtracted from the selling price.

Points to Remember:

- The face value of a share always remains the same.
- The market value of a share changes from time to time.
- Dividend is always paid on the face value of a share.
- Number of shares held by a person

$$\frac{\text{Total Investment}}{\text{Investment in one share}} = \frac{\text{Total Income}}{\text{Income from one share}} = \frac{\text{Total Face Value}}{\text{Face of one share}}$$

② Algebra Formulae

SURDS AND INDICES

Law of Indices

If x and y are two positive real numbers and n and m are two positive integers ($n > m$) then,

(i) $\dfrac{x^n}{x^m} = x^{n-m}$

(ii) $x^n x^m = x^{n+m}$

(iii) $x^n y^n = (xy)^n$

(iv) $\left[\dfrac{x}{y}\right]^n = \dfrac{x^n}{y^n}$

(v) $\left[\dfrac{x}{y}\right]^{-n} = \left[\dfrac{y}{x}\right]^n$

(vi) $x^{-n} = \dfrac{1}{x^n}$

(vii) $(x^y)^z = x^{(y \times z)}$

(viii) $x^\circ = 1$

An irrational nth root (square, cube or higher) which cannot be expressed as a common fraction is known as surd.

If a is a positive rational number and n is a positive integer such that

$a^{\frac{1}{n}} = \sqrt[n]{a}$, then

(i) $\sqrt[n]{a}$ is called surd or radical.

(ii) n is called the order of the surd.

(iii) a is called the radicand.

Law of Surds

For positive real numbers x, y, a, b and natural numbers m and n :

(i) $\sqrt{x} \times \sqrt{y} = \sqrt{xy}$

(ii) $\sqrt{x} \times \sqrt{x} = x$

(iii) $\sqrt{\dfrac{x}{y}} = \dfrac{\sqrt{x}}{\sqrt{y}}$

       Mathematics Formulae

(iv) $\left[\sqrt{x}\right]^{n} = \sqrt{x^{n}}$

(v) $\sqrt[m]{x^{n}} = x^{\frac{n}{m}}$

(vi) $a\sqrt{c} + b\sqrt{c} = (a+b)\sqrt{c}$

(vii) $\sqrt{a} + \sqrt{b} \neq \sqrt{a+b}$

(viii) $\sqrt{a} + \sqrt{a} = 2\sqrt{a}$

(ix) $a\sqrt{c} - b\sqrt{c} = (a-b)\sqrt{c}$

(x) $\left(\sqrt{a} + \sqrt{b}\right)\left(\sqrt{a} - \sqrt{b}\right) = a - b$

(xi) $\left(a + \sqrt{b}\right)\left(a - \sqrt{b}\right) = a^{2} - b$

(xii) $a^{\frac{x}{y}} = \sqrt[y]{a^{x}}$

(xiii) $\left(\sqrt[n]{a}\right)^{n} = a$

(xiv) If $a^{m} = b^{m}$, then $a = b$

(xv) If $a^{m} = a^{n}$, then $m = n$

Note: If x and y are negative real numbers, then $\sqrt{x} \times \sqrt{y} \neq \sqrt{xy}$

Rationalizing Surd

Rationalizing the surd is the process of getting rid of the surd in the denominator of a fraction.

> To rationalize, we multiply the numerator and denominator by a fraction which equals one.
>
> To rationalize fractions in the form $\sqrt{\dfrac{1}{a}}$, multiply the numerator and denominator by $\sqrt{a}$
>
> To rationalize fractions in the form $\dfrac{1}{a+\sqrt{b}}$, multiply the numerator and denominator by $a - \sqrt{b}$
>
> To rationalize fractions in the form $\dfrac{1}{a-\sqrt{b}}$, multiply the numerator and denominator by $a + \sqrt{b}$

VARIATION

Direct Proportion

Two quantities x and y are said to be in direct proportion if they increase (decrease) together in such a manner that the ratio of their corresponding values remains constant.

In other words two quantities x and y vary directly if $\dfrac{x}{y} = k$ where k is a positive number.

If y_1, y_2 are the values of y corresponding to the values x_1, x_2 of x respectively, then $\dfrac{x_1}{y_1} = \dfrac{x_2}{y_2}$

Note: When two quantities x and y are in direct proportion (or vary directly) they are also written as $x \quad y$.

Inverse Proportion

Two quantities x and y are said to be in inverse proportion if an increase in x causes a proportional decrease in y (and vice-versa) in such a manner that the product of their corresponding values remains constant.

That is, if $xy = k$, then x and y are said to vary inversely.

If y_1, y_2 are the values of y corresponding to the values x_1, x_2 of x respectively, then

$x_1 y_1 = x_2 y_2$ or $\dfrac{x_1}{x_2} = \dfrac{y_2}{y_1}$

Note: When two quantities x and y are in inverse proportion (or vary indirectly) they are also written as $x \propto \dfrac{1}{y}$.

POLYNOMIAL

Polynomial

A polynomial *p(x)* in one variable x is an algebraic expression in x of the form

$p(x) = a_n x^n + a_{n-1} x^{n-1} + \quad + a_2 x^2 + a_1 x + a_0$,

where a_0, a_1, a_2,...,a_n are constants and a_n

a_0, a_1, a_2,..., a_n $\hspace{3cm}$ x^0, x^1, x^2,...,x^n, and '*n*' is known as the degree of the polynomial. Each of $a_n x^n$, ..., $a_0 x^0$ is called a term of the polynomial.

Monomial : A polynomial of one term is called a monomial.

Binomial : A polynomial of two terms is called a binomial.

Trinomial : A polynomial of three terms is called a trinomial.

Linear Polynomial

A polynomial of degree one is called a linear polynomial.

The zero of a linear polynomial $\hspace{2cm}$ is given by

$$\dfrac{-b}{a} = \dfrac{-(\text{Constant term})}{\text{Coefficient of } x}$$

- For a linear polynomial $ax + b$, $a \neq 0$, the graph of $y = ax + b$ is a straight line which intersects the x-axis at exactly one point, $\left(\dfrac{-b}{a}, 0\right)$.

Therefore, the linear polynomial $ax + b$, $a \neq 0$, has exactly one zero, the x-coordinate of the point where the graph of $y = ax + b$ intersects the x-axis.

Quadratic Polynomial
A polynomial of degree two is called a quadratic polynomial.
- A quadratic polynomial in x with real coefficients is of the form $ax^2 + bx + c$, where a, b, c are real numbers with $a \neq 0$.
- A quadratic polynomial can have at most 2 zeroes. It can have either two distinct zeroes or two equal zeroes or no zero.
- If α and β are the zeroes of the quadratic polynomial $ax^2 + bx + c$, then $\alpha + \beta = -\dfrac{b}{a}, \alpha\beta = \dfrac{c}{a}$
- The graph of $ax^2 + bx + c$, where a, b, c are real numbers and $a \neq 0$ is a parabola.

Cubic Polynomial
A polynomial of degree three is called a cubic polynomial.
- A cubic polynomial in x with real coefficients is of the form, $ax^3 + bx^2 + cx + d = 0$ where a, b, c, d are real numbers with $a \neq 0$.
- A cubic polynomial can have at most 3 zeroes.
- If α, β, γ are the zeroes of the cubic polynomial $ax^3 + bx^2 + cx + d = 0$, then

$$\alpha + \beta + \gamma = \dfrac{-b}{a},$$

$$\alpha\beta + \beta\gamma + \gamma\alpha = \dfrac{c}{a},$$

$$\text{and } \alpha\beta\gamma = \dfrac{-d}{a}$$

Constant Polynomial
A polynomial without any variable or variable with power zero is called a constant polynomial. For example, $p(x) = 8$, $x^0 [x^0 = 1]$. The degree of a non-zero constant polynomial is zero.

Zero polynomial
The constant polynomial 0 is called a zero polynomial. The degree of a zero polynomial is not defined.

Zero of a polynomial
A real number 'a' is a zero of a polynomial $p(x)$ if $p(a) = 0$. In this case, a is also called a root of the equation $p(x) = 0$.

- Every linear polynomial in one variable has a unique zero.
- A non-zero constant polynomial has no zero.
- Every real number is a zero of the zero polynomial.
- The zeroes of a polynomial $p(x)$ are precisely the x-coordinates of the points, where the graph of $y = p(x)$ intersects the x-axis.

Graph of a Polynomial

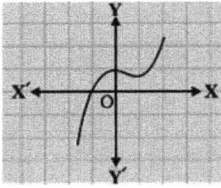
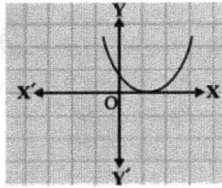
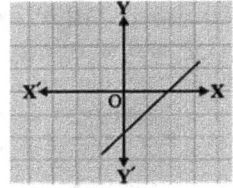

One zero

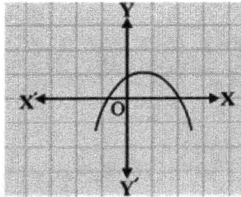
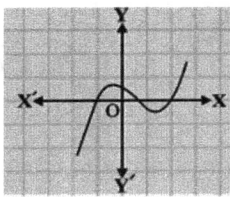
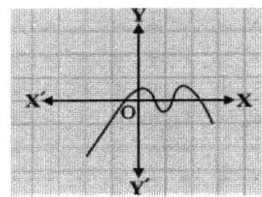

Two zeroes   Three zeroes   Four zeroes

Division Algorithm of a Polynomial

If $p(x)$ and $g(x)$ are two polynomials such that degree of $p(x) \geq$ degree of $g(x)$ and $g(x) \neq 0$, then we can find polynomials $q(x)$ and $r(x)$ such that:

$$p(x) = g(x)q(x) + r(x),$$

where

$$r(x) = 0 \text{ or degree of } r(x) < \text{degree of } g(x).$$

Hence, $p(x)$ divided by $g(x)$ gives quotient as $q(x)$ and remainder as $r(x)$.

Remainder Theorem

If $p(x)$ is any polynomial of degree greater than or equal to 1 and $p(x)$ is divided by the linear polynomial $x - a$, then the remainder is $p(a)$.

Factor Theorem

$x - a$ is a factor of the polynomial $p(x)$, if $p(a) = 0$. Also, if $x - a$ is a factor of $p(x)$, then $p(a) = 0$.

PARTIAL FRACTION

Rational Fraction

A fraction in which both the numerator and the denominator are polynomials and the denominator is not equal to zero is called a rational fraction.

Proper Rational Fraction

If the degree of the numerator of a rational fraction is less than the degree of the denominator of the rational fraction, then that fraction is known as a proper rational fraction.

Improper Rational Fraction

If the degree of the numerator of the rational fraction is greater than the degree of the denominator of the rational fraction, then that fraction is known as an improper rational fraction.

Partial Fraction Expansion

Partial fraction expansion or partial fraction decomposition of a rational fraction is the proces by which the rational fraction can be expressed as a sum of a polynomial and one or more fractions with a simple denominator.

Steps for Solving Partial Fraction

(i) If $\dfrac{P(x)}{Q(x)}$ is an improper rational function, divide $P(x)$ by $Q(x)$.

$\dfrac{P(x)}{Q(x)} = T(x) + \dfrac{R(x)}{Q(x)}$ where $T(x)$ is the quotient and $R(x)$ is the remainder.

(ii) Write $\dfrac{R(x)}{Q(x)}$ as partial fraction expansion.

(iii) Simplify.

Partial Fraction Expansion of Some Common Rational Fractions

If A, B, C and D are real numbers then:

S.No.	Rational Fraction	Partial Fraction Expansion
1.	$\dfrac{px+q}{(x-a)(x-b)}$,	$\dfrac{A}{(x-a)}+\dfrac{B}{(x-b)}$
2.	$\dfrac{px+q}{(x-a)^2}$	$\dfrac{A}{(x-a)}+\dfrac{B}{(x-a)^2}$
3.	$\dfrac{px+q}{(x-a)^3}$	$\dfrac{A}{(x-a)}+\dfrac{B}{(x-a)^2}+\dfrac{C}{(x-a)^3}$
4.	$\dfrac{px^2+qx+r}{(x-a)(x-b)(x-c)}$	$\dfrac{A}{(x-a)}+\dfrac{B}{(x-b)}+\dfrac{C}{(x-c)}$
5.	$\dfrac{px^2+qx+r}{(x-a)^2(x-b)}$	$\dfrac{A}{(x-a)}+\dfrac{B}{(x-a)^2}+\dfrac{C}{(x-b)}$
6.	$\dfrac{px^2+qx+r}{(x-a)^3(x-b)}$	$\dfrac{A}{(x-a)}+\dfrac{B}{(x-a)^2}+\dfrac{C}{(x-a)^3}+\dfrac{D}{(x-b)}$
7.	$\dfrac{px^2+qx+r}{(x-a)(x^2+bx+c)}$	$\dfrac{A}{(x-a)}+\dfrac{Bx+C}{x^2+bx+c}$, where x^2+bx+c can not be factored further

ALGEBRAIC IDENTITY

Square of a Binomial

$(a+b)^2 = a^2 + 2ab + b^2$

$(a-b)^2 = a^2 - 2ab + b^2$

Difference of Squares

$a^2 \quad b^2 = (a+b)(a \quad b)$

Sum of Squares
$(a^2 + b^2) = (a + b)^2 - 2ab$

Product of Binomials
$(x + a)(x + b) = x^2 + (a + b)x + ab$

Cube of a Binomial
$(a + b)^3 = a^3 + 3 \cdot a^2 \cdot b + 3 \cdot a \cdot b^2 + b^3$
$(\quad)^3 = a^3 \qquad {}^2 \cdot b + 3 \cdot a \cdot b^2 \qquad {}^3$

Square of a Trinomial
$(a + b + c)^2 = a^2 + b^2 + c^2 + 2 \cdot a \cdot b + 2 \cdot b \cdot c + 2 \cdot a \cdot c$

Sum of Cubes
$a^3 + b^3 = (a + b)(a^2 \quad ab + b^2)$

Difference of Cubes
$a^3 \quad b^3 = (a \quad b)(a^2 + ab + b^2)$

Fourth Power of a Binomial
$(a + b)^4 = (a + b)^3(a + b) = a^4 + 4a^3b + 6a^2b^2 + 4ab^3 + b^4$

Sum of Fourth Power
$a^4 + b^4 = (a^2 - \sqrt{2} \cdot a \cdot b + b^2)(a^2 + \sqrt{2} \cdot a \cdot b + b^2)$

Difference of Fourth Power
$a^4 - b^4 = (a^2 - b^2)(a^2 + b^2) = (a + b)(a - b)(a^2 + b^2)$

Sum of Fifth Power
$a^5 + b^5 = (a + b)(a^4 - a^3b + a^2b^2 - ab^3 + b^4)$

Difference of Fifth Power
$a^5 - b^5 = (a - b)(a^4 + a^3b + a^2b^2 + ab^3 + b^4)$

Sum of nth Power
$a^n + b^n = (a + b)(a^{n-1} - ba^{n-2} + b^2a^{n-3} - \ldots - b^{n-2}a + b^{n-1})$

Difference of nth Power
$a^n - b^n = (a - b)(a^{n-1} + ba^{n-2} + b^2a^{n-3} + \ldots + b^{n-2}a + b^{n-1})$

Another Important Identity
$a^3 + b^3 + c^3 \quad abc = (a + b + c)(a^2 + b^2 + c^2 - ab - bc - ca)$

EQUALITY AND INEQUALITY

Properties of Equality
If A and B are algebraic expressions and c is a real number then,

Addition Property of Equality
If A = B, then A + c = B + c

Subtraction Property of Equality
If $A = B$, then $A - c = B - c$

Multiplication Property of Equality
If $A = B$ and $c \neq 0$, then $cA = cB$

Division Property of Equality
If $A = B$ and $c \neq 0$, then $\dfrac{A}{c} = \dfrac{B}{c}$

Note:
- Multiplying or dividing both sides of an equation by zero is avoided.
- Division by zero is undefined and multiplying both sides by zero will result in an equation $0 = 0$.

Symmetric Property
If $A = B$, then $B = A$

Transitive Property
If $A = B$ and $B = C$, then $A = C$

Definition of Inequality
Two real numbers or two algebraic expressions related by the symbols $<, >, \leq$ or $\geq$ form an inequality.

Rules of Inequality
(i) Equal numbers may be added to (or subtracted from) both sides of an inequality.

If $a > b$, then $a + c > b + c$

If $a < b$, then $a + c < b + c$

(ii) Both sides of an inequality can be multiplied (or divided) by the same positive number.

If $a > b$ and $c > 0$, then $ac > bc$

If $a > b$ and $c > 0$, then $\dfrac{a}{c} > \dfrac{b}{c}$

(iii) When both sides of an inequality are multiplied (or divided) by a negative number, then the inequality is reversed.

If $a > b$ and $c < 0$, then $ac < bc$

If $a > b$ and $c < 0$, then $\dfrac{a}{c} < \dfrac{b}{c}$

(iv) For double inequalities:

If $a > b$ and $c > d$, then $a + c > b + d$

If $a > b$ and $c = d$, then $a + c > b + d$

If $a < b$ and $c < d$, then $a + c < b + d$

If $a < b$ and $c = d$, then $a + c < b + d$

The values of x, which makes an inequality a true statement, are called solutions of the inequality.

Number Line of an Inequality

To represent $x < a$ (or $x > a$) on a number line, put a dark circle on the number on a and dark line to the left (or right) of the number a.

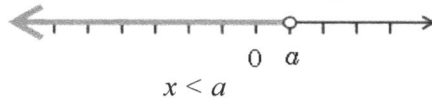

$$x < a$$

To represent (or) on a number line, put a dark circle on the number on a and dark line to the left (or right) of the number x.

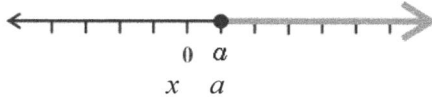

$$x \quad a$$

Graph of an Inequality

symbol, then the points on the line are also included in the solutions of the inequality and the graph of the inequality lies left (below) or right (above) of the graph of the equality

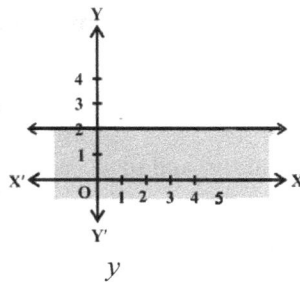

$$y$$

an arbitrary point in that part.

If an inequality is having $<$ or $>$ symbol, then the points on the line are not included in the solutions of the inequality and the graph of the inequality lies to the left (below) or right (above) of the graph of the corresponding equality represented

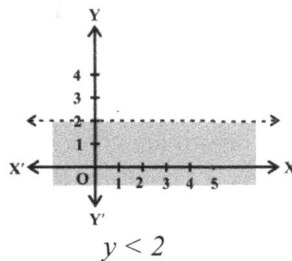

$$y < 2$$

arbitrary point in that part.

The region containing all the solutions of an inequality is called the solution region.

LINEAR EQUATION

Equation

An equation is a statement indicating that two algebraic expressions are equal.

Linear Equation in One Variable

A linear equation in one variable x is an equation that can be written in the form $ax + b = 0$ where a and b are real numbers and a

Solution of a Linear Equation

The solution of a linear equation is not affected when:

(i) the same number is added to (or subtracted from) both sides of the equation.

(ii) the same non-zero number is multiplied or divided by on both sides of the equation.

(iii)A linear equation in one variable has only one solution.

Linear Equation in Two Variables

An equation of the form $ax + by + c = 0$, where a, b and c are real numbers, such that a and b both are not zero, is called a linear equation in two variables.

Solution of Linear Equations in Two Variables

A linear equation in two variables has infinitely many solutions.

Each solution (x, y) of a linear equation in two variables,

$ax + by + c = 0$, corresponds to a point on the line representing the equation, and vice versa.

$x = 0$ is the equation of the y-axis and $y = 0$ is the equation of the x-axis.

Graph of Linear Equations in Two Variables

- The graph of every linear equation in two variables is a straight line.
- The graph of $x = a$ is a straight line parallel to the y-axis.
- The graph of $y = a$ is a straight line parallel to the x-axis.
- An equation of the type $y = mx$ represents a line passing through the origin.
- Every point on the graph of a linear equation in two variables is a solution of the linear equation. Every solution of the linear equation is a point on the graph of the linear equation.

Pair of Linear Equations in Two Variables

Two linear equations in the same two variables are called a pair of linear equations in two variables. The most general form of a pair of linear equations is

$$a_1 x + b_1 y + c_1 = 0$$
$$a_2 x + b_2 y + c_2 = 0$$

where a_1, a_2, b_1, b_2, c_1, c_2 are real numbers, such that

$$a_1^2 + b_1^2 \neq 0, \quad a_2^2 + b_2^2 \neq 0.$$

Solution of a pair of linear equations

A pair of linear equations in two variables can be represented and solved by the following methods.

(a) Graphical method

The graph of a pair of linear equations in two variables is represented by two lines.

(i) If the lines intersect at a point, then that point gives the unique solution of the two equations. The pair of equations is said to be consistent in this case.

(ii) If the lines coincide, then there are infinitely many solutions — each point on the line being a solution. In this case, the pair of equations is dependent (Dependent equations are always consistent).

(iii) If the lines are parallel, then the pair of equations has no solution. The pair of equations is said to be inconsistent in this case.

(b) Algebraic method

Different methods for solving a pair of linear equations by algebraic methods are:

(i) *Substitution Method*

• Find the value of one variable in terms of the other variable from one of the equations (*i.e.* x in terms of y).

• Substitute this value of the variable in the other equation, and reduce it to an equation in one variable. Solve it.

• Now substitute the value of the variable obtained in second step in the equation used in the first step to obtain the other variable.

(ii) *Elimination Method*

• Multiply both the equations by some suitable non-zero constant to make the coefficient of one of the variables numerically equal.

• Next add or subtract one equation from the other in order to eliminate one of the variables.

If we get an equation in one variable, go to the third step.

If in the second step, we get a true statement involving no variable, then the original pair of equations has infinitely many solutions.

If in the second step, we get a false statement involving no variable, then the original pair of equations has no solution,

• Solve the equation in one variable.

• Substitute this value of the variable in either of the original equations to get the value of the other variable.

(iii) Cross-multiplication Method

If a pair of linear equations is given by

$$a_1x + b_1y + c_1 = 0$$

$$a_2x + b_2y + c_2 = 0$$

then

$$x = \frac{b_1c_2 - b_2c_1}{a_1b_2 - a_2b_1}, y = \frac{c_1a_2 - c_2a_1}{a_1b_2 - a_2b_1} \text{ provided } a_1b_1 - a_2b_2$$

Different Conditions

If a pair of linear equations is given by

$$a_1x + b_1y + c_1 = 0$$

$$a_2x + b_2y + c_2 = 0$$

then the following situations can arise :

(i) $\frac{a_1}{a_2} \neq \frac{b_1}{b_2}$

In this case, the pair of linear equations is consistent.

(ii) $\frac{a_1}{a_2} = \frac{b_1}{b_2} \neq \frac{c_1}{c_2}$

In this case, the pair of linear equations is inconsistent.

(iii) $\frac{a_1}{a_2} = \frac{b_1}{b_2} = \frac{c_1}{c_2}$

In this case, the pair of linear equations is consistent and dependent.

AGE PROBLEMS

While solving age problems, represent the following in terms of a variable:

(i) the present ages of people, animals etc.

Then, form an equation based on the variables as per the given conditions.

Main Rules

(i) If the present age is x, then n times the age is nx

(ii) If the present age is x, then age n years later/hence $= x + n$

(iii) If the present age is x, then age n years ago $= x - n$

(iv) The ages in a ratio $a : b$ will be ax and bx

(v) If the present age is x, then $\frac{1}{n}$ of the age is $\frac{x}{n}$

QUADRATIC EQUATION

Standard Form of Quadratic Equation

An equation of degree two is known as a quadratic equation. The general form or standard form of a quadratic equation is $ax^2 + bx + c = 0$, where x represents a variable or an unknown, and a, b, and c are constants with a $a = 0$, the equation is reduced to a linear equation).

Roots of a Quadratic Equation

$$ax^2 + bx + c = 0, \text{ if } a\ ^2 + b\ \ + c = 0,$$

$ax^2 + bx + c$ and the roots of the quadratic equation $ax^2 + bx + c = 0$ are the same.

$$ax^2 + bx + c,\ a$$

two linear factors, then the roots of the quadratic equation $ax^2 + bx + c = 0$ can be found by equating each factor to zero.

Completing Square

(i) Write the quadratic equation in the standard form.

(ii) Divide each side by a

(iii) Rearrange the equation so that the constant term $\frac{c}{a}$ is on the right side.

(iv) Add the square of half of $\frac{b}{a}$ x, to both sides. This completes the square, converting the left side into a perfect square.

(v) Write the left side as a perfect square and simplify the right side if required.

(vi) Make two linear equations by equating the square root of the left side with the positive and negative square roots of the right side.

(vii) Solve the two linear equations.

Quadratic Formula

The two roots of the quadratic equation ax^2 are given by

$$x_1 = \frac{-b + \sqrt{b^2 - 4ac}}{2a}, \ x_2 = \frac{-b - \sqrt{b^2 - 4ac}}{2a} \text{ provided } b^2 - 4ac$$

$b^2 - 4ac$ is called the discriminant of the quadratic equation $ax^2 + bx + c = 0$.

Nature of Roots

If $b^2 - 4ac > 0$, the equation has two real and distinct roots.

If $b^2 - 4ac = 0$, both the roots are real and equal.

If $b^2 - 4ac < 0$, the roots are complex conjugate.

Graph of Quadratic Polynomial

The graph of quadratic polynomial ax^2 is given by

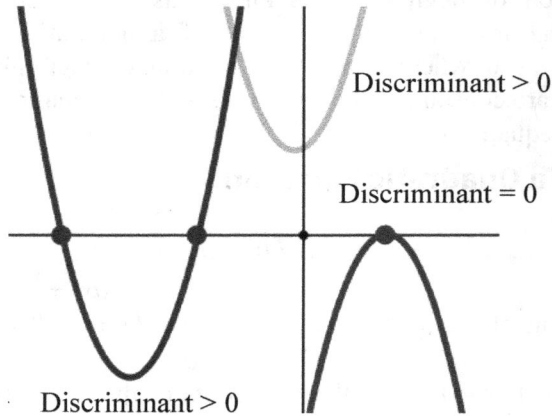

Discriminant > 0

Discriminant = 0

Discriminant > 0

Sum and Product of Roots

Sum of roots of a quadratic equation $= \dfrac{-b}{a}$

Product of roots of a quadratic equation $= \dfrac{c}{a}$

When both sum and product of the roots of a quadratic equation are given, the equation is determined by using the formula:

$$x^2 - (\text{sum of roots})x + \text{Product of roots} = 0$$

COMPLEX NUMBER

A number of the form $a + ib$, where a and b are real numbers, is called a complex number, a is called the real part and b is called the imaginary part of the complex number. A complex number is generally represented by the letter Z.

Equality of Complex Numbers

Two complex numbers $a + ib$ and $c + id$ are said to be equal if $a = c$ and $b = d$.

Sum of Complex Numbers

Let $z_1 = a + ib$ and $z_2 = c + id$. Then

$$z_1 + z_2 = (a + c) + i\,(b + d)$$

Addition Properties of Complex Numbers

(i) Closure Law
The sum of two complex numbers is a complex number, i.e., $z_1 + z_2$ is a complex number for all complex numbers z_1 and z_2.

(ii) Commutative Law
For any two complex numbers z_1 and z_2, $z_1 + z_2 = z_2 + z_1$

(iii) Associative Law
For any three complex numbers z_1, z_2 and z_3,
$$(z_1 + z_2) + z_3 = z_1 + (z_2 + z_3)$$

(iv) Additive Identity
There exists the complex number $0 + i\,0$, called the additive identity such that, for every complex number z, $z + 0 = z$

(v) Additive Inverse
For every complex number $z = a + ib$, the complex number $-a + i(-b)$ (denoted as $-z$), is known as the additive inverse .
$$z + (-z) = 0$$

Difference of Complex Numbers
Let $z_1 = a + ib$ and $z_2 = c + id$. Then $z_1 - z_2 = z_1 + (-z_2) = (a - c) + i(b - d)$

Product of Complex Numbers
Let $z_1 = a + ib$ and $z_2 = c + id$. Then $z_1 z_2 = (ac - bd) + i(ad + bc)$

Multiplication Properties of Complex Numbers

(i) Closure Law
The product of two complex numbers is a complex number, i.e., $z_1 z_2$ is a complex number for all complex numbers z_1 and z_2

(ii) Commutative Law
For any two complex numbers z_1 and z_2, $z_1 z_2 = z_2 z_1$

(iii) Associative Law
For any three complex numbers z_1, z_2 and z_3, $(z_1 z_2) z_3 = z_1 (z_2 z_3)$

(iv) Multiplicative Identity
There exists the complex number $1 + i\,0$, called the multiplicative identity such that, for every complex number z, $z.1 = z$

(v) Multiplicative Inverse
For any non-zero complex number $z = a + ib$ ($a \neq 0,\ b \neq 0$), there exists the complex number $\dfrac{a}{a^2 + b^2} + i\dfrac{-b}{a^2 + b^2}$ denoted by z^{-1} which is known as the multiplicative inverse of z such that
$$(a + ib)\left(\frac{a}{a^2 + b^2} + i\frac{-b}{a^2 + b^2} \right) = 1 + i0 = 1$$

(vi) Distributive Property

For any three complex numbers z_1, z_2 and z_3, $z_1 (z_2 + z_3) = z_1 z_2 + z_1 z_3$, $(z_1 + z_2) z_3 = z_1 z_3 + z_2 z_3$

Quotient of Complex Numbers

Let $z_1 = a + ib$ and $z_2 = c + id$. Then if $z_2 \neq 0$, the quotient is defined by $\dfrac{z_1}{z_2} = z_1 \dfrac{1}{z_2}$

Power of i

$i^2 = -1$ and $(-i)^2 = i^2 = -1$

$i^3 = i^2 i = (-1)i = -i$

$i^4 = (i^2)^2 = (-1)^2 = 1$

$i^5 = (i^2)^2 i = (-1)^2 i = i$

$i^{-1} = \dfrac{1}{i} \times \dfrac{i}{i} = \dfrac{i}{-1} = -i$

$i^{-2} = \dfrac{1}{i^2} = \dfrac{1}{-1} = -1$

For any integer k, $i^{4k} = 1$, $i^{4k+1} = i$, $i^{4k+2} = -1$, $i^{4k+3} = -i$

Identities in Complex Numbers

For all complex numbers $z_1 = a + ib$ and $z_2 = c + id$,

(i) $(z_1 + z_2)^2 = z_1^2 + z_2^2 + 2z_1 z_2$

(ii) $(z_1 - z_2)^2 = z_1^2 - 2z_1 z_2 + z_2^2$

(iii) $(z_1 + z_2)^3 = z_1^3 + 3z_1^2 z_2 + 3z_1 z_2^2 + z_2^3$

(iv) $(z_1 - z_2)^3 = z_1^3 - 3z_1^2 z_2 + 3z_1 z_2^2 - z_2^3$

(v) $z_1^2 - z_2^2 = (z_1 + z_2)(z_1 - z_2)$

Modulus of a Complex Number

The modulus of the complex number $z = a + ib$ is denoted by $|Z|$. It is defined as

$$|z| = \sqrt{a^2 + b^2}$$

Conjugate of a Complex Number

The conjugate of a complex number $z = a + ib$ denoted by $\bar{z}$ is given by $a - ib$.

Relation between Multiplicative Inverse and Modulus of a Complex Number

For the complex number $z = a + ib$,

$$z^{-1} = \frac{\bar{z}}{|z|^2} \text{ or } z\bar{z} = |z|^2$$

Properties of Modulus of Complex Number

For any two complex numbers, $z_1 = a + ib$ and $z_2 = c + id$,

(i) $|z_1 z_2| = |z_1||z_2|$

(ii) $\left|\dfrac{z_1}{z_2}\right| = \dfrac{|z_1|}{|z_2|}$ provided $|z_2| \neq 0$

(iii) $\overline{z_1 z_2} = \overline{z_1}\,\overline{z_2}$

(iv) $\overline{z_1 + z_2} = \overline{z_1} + \overline{z_2}$

(v) $\overline{z_1 - z_2} = \overline{z_1} - \overline{z_2}$

(vi) $\overline{\left(\dfrac{z_1}{z_2}\right)} = \dfrac{\overline{z_1}}{\overline{z_2}}$ provided $z_2 \neq 0$

Argand Diagram

An Argand diagram is a plot of complex numbers as points in the Argand plane. The real part of the number is plotted along the horizontal axis (x-axis) and the imaginary part is plotted along the vertical axis (y-axis).

In the Argand plane, the modulus of the complex number $z = a + ib$ is the distance between the origin and the point $A(a, b)$.

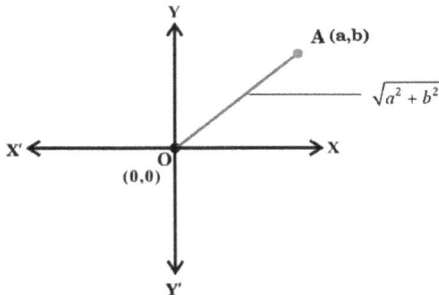

Polar Form of a Complex Number

The polar form of the complex number $z = x + iy$ is $r(\cos\theta + i\sin\theta)$, where $r = \sqrt{x^2 + y^2}$ (the modulus of z) and $\cos\theta = \dfrac{x}{r}, \sin\theta = \dfrac{y}{r}$ (θ is the angle which the directed line segment of length r makes with the positive direction of x axis. It is known as the argument of z).

- For any complex number $z \neq 0$, there is only one value of θ in $0 \leq \theta < 2\pi$

- The value of θ such that $-\pi < \theta \leq \pi$ is called the principal argument of z

$0 \leq \theta < 2\pi$

$-\pi < \theta \leq \pi$

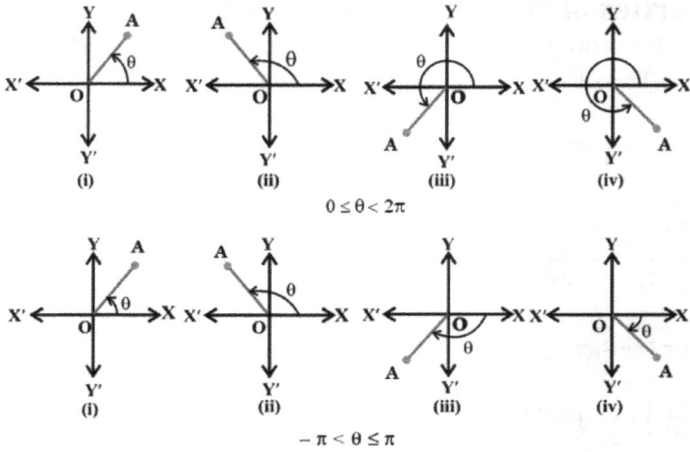

Fundamental Theorem of Algebra

A polynomial equation has at least one root. A polynomial equation of n degree has n roots.

The roots of the quadratic equation ax^2
$b^2 - 4ac < 0$ are given by

$$x = \frac{-b \pm \sqrt{4ac - b^2}\, i}{2a}$$

MATRICES

A matrix is an ordered rectangular array of numbers or functions. The numbers or functions are called the elements or entries of the matrix. A matrix is denoted by a capital letter.

A matrix having m rows and n columns is called a matrix of order $m \times n$.

$$\begin{bmatrix} a_{11} & a_{12} & a_{13} \cdots a_{1j} \cdots a_{1n} \\ a_{21} & a_{22} & a_{23} \cdots a_{2j} \cdots a_{2n} \\ a_{r1} & a_{r2} & a_{r3} \cdots a_{ij} \cdots a_{in} \\ a_{m1} & a_{m2} & a_{m3} \cdots a_{mj} \cdots a_{mn} \end{bmatrix}_{m \times n}$$

The number of elements in $m \times n$ matrix is equal to mn.

Types of matrices
Column Matrix
A matrix is said to be a column matrix if it has only one column. $[a_{ij}]_{m \times 1}$ is a column matrix of order $m \times 1$.

Row Matrix

A matrix is said to be a row matrix if it has only one row. $[a_{ij}]_{1 \times n}$ is a row matrix of order $1 \times n$

Square Matrix

A matrix is said to be a square matrix if the number of rows are equal to the number of columns. An $m \times n$ matrix is a square matrix if $m = n$. It is of order n.

Diagonal Matrix

A square matrix $A = [a_{ij}]_{m \times m}$ is a diagonal matrix if all its non diagonal elements are zero i.e. $a_{ij} = 0$, when $i \neq j$

Scalar Matrix

A diagonal matrix is said to be a scalar matrix if its diagonal elements are equal. $A = [a_{ij}]_{n \times n}$ is a scalar matrix if $a_{ij} = 0$, when $i \neq j$, $a_{ij} = k$, (k is some constant), when $i = j$.

Identity Matrix

A square matrix in which the elements in the diagonal are all 1 and rest are all zero is called an identity matrix.

$A = [a_{ij}]_{n \times n}$ is an identity matrix, if $a_{ij} = 1$, when $i = j$ and $a_{ij} = 0$, when $i \neq j$.

Zero Matrix

A zero matrix or null matrix has all its elements as zero.

Equality of Matrices

$A = [a_{ij}] = [b_{ij}] = B$ if

  (i) A and B are of same order,

  (ii) $a_{ij} = b_{ij}$ for all possible values of i and j.

Operations on Matrices
Addition of Matrices

If $A = \begin{bmatrix} a_{11} & a_{12} & a_{13} \\ a_{21} & a_{22} & a_{23} \end{bmatrix}$ is a 2×3 matrix and $B = \begin{bmatrix} b_{11} & b_{12} & b_{13} \\ b_{21} & b_{22} & b_{23} \end{bmatrix}$ is another

2×3 matrix, then the sum of two matrices is defined by

$$A + B = \begin{bmatrix} a_{11}+b_{11} & a_{12}+b_{12} & a_{13}+b_{13} \\ a_{21}+b_{21} & a_{22}+b_{22} & a_{23}+b_{23} \end{bmatrix}$$

If $A = [a_{ij}]$ and $B = [b_{ij}]$ are two matrices of the same order, i.e. $m \times n$, then the sum of two matrices A and B is defined as a matrix $C = [c_{ij}]_{m \times n}$, where $c_{ij} = a_{ij} + b_{ij}$, for all possible values of i and j.

Note: If A and B are not of the same order, then $A + B$ is not defined.

Multiplication of a Matrix by a Scalar
If $A = [a_{ij}]_{m \times n}$ is a matrix and k is a scalar, then kA is another matrix which is obtained by multiplying each element of A by the scalar k.
$$kA = k[a_{ij}]_{m \times n} = [k(a_{ij})]_{m \times n}$$

Negative of a Matrix
The negative of a matrix is defined by $-A$.
$$-A = (-1)A$$

Difference of Matrices
If $A = [a_{ij}]$, $B = [b_{ij}]$ are two matrices of the same order, i.e. $m \times n$, then the difference $A - B$ is defined as a matrix $D = [d_{ij}]$, where $d_{ij} = a_{ij} - b_{ij}$, for all values of i and j.
In other words, $A - B = A + (-1) B$, that is sum of the matrix A and the matrix $- B$.

Properties of Matrix Addition

(i) Commutative Law
If $A = [a_{ij}]$, $B = [b_{ij}]$ are matrices of the same order, i.e. $m \times n$, then
$$A + B = B + A$$

(ii) Associative Law
For any three matrices $A = [a_{ij}]$, $B = [b_{ij}]$, $C = [c_{ij}]$ of the same order, i.e. $m \times n$, $(A + B) + C = A + (B + C)$

(iii) Existence of additive identity
Let $A = [a_{ij}]$ be an $m \times n$ matrix and O be an $m \times n$ zero matrix, then $A + O = O + A = A$. In other words, O is the additive identity for matrix addition.

(iv) Additive Inverse
Let $A = [a_{ij}]_{m \times n}$ be any matrix, then we have another matrix as $- A = [- a_{ij}]_{m \times n}$ such that $A + (- A) = (- A) + A = O$. So $- A$ is the additive inverse of A or negative of A.

# Properties of Scalar Multiplication of a Matrix
If $A = [a_{ij}]$ and $B = [b_{ij}]$ be two matrices of the same order, i.e. $m \times n$ and k and l are scalars, then
 (i) $k(A + B) = kA + kB$
 (ii) $(k + l)A = k A + l A$

Product of Matrices
The product of two matrices A and B is defined if the number of columns of A is equal to the number of rows of B.
Let $A = [a_{ij}]$ be an $m \times n$ matrix and $B = [b_{jk}]$ be an $n \times p$ matrix. Then the product of the matrices A and B is the matrix C of order $m \times p$.

If $A = [a_{ij}]_{m \times n}$, $B = [b_{jk}]_{n \times p}$, then the ith row of A is $[a_{i1} \ a_{i2} \ \ldots \ a_{in}]$ and the

k^{th} column of B is $\begin{bmatrix} b_{1k} \\ b_{2k} \\ \vdots \\ b_{nk} \end{bmatrix}$, then

$$c_{ik} = a_{i1}b_{1k} + a_{i2}b_{2k} + a_{i3}b_{3k} + \ldots + a_{in}b_{nk} = \sum_{j=1}^{n} a_{ij}b_{jk}$$

The matrix $C = [c_{ik}]_{m \times p}$ is the product of A and B.

Properties of Matrix Multiplication

If A, B and C are $m \times n$, $n \times p$ and $m \times p$ matrices respectively, then:

(i) Associative Law
(AB) C = A (BC), whenever both sides of the equality are defined.

(ii) Distributive Law
(a) A (B + C) = AB + AC

(b) (A + B) C = AC + BC, whenever both sides of equality are defined.

(iii) Existence of Multiplicative Identity
For every square matrix A, there exists an identity matrix of same order such that IA = AI = A

Note:

- Matrix multiplication is not always commutative i.e. AB ≠ BA even if both AB and BA are defined.
- If the product of two matrices is a zero matrix, it is not necessary that one of the matrix is a zero matrix.

Transpose of a Matrix

If $A = [a_{ij}]$ be an $m \times n$ matrix, then the matrix obtained by interchanging the rows and columns of A is called the transpose of A. Transpose of the matrix A is denoted by A' or (A^T).

In other words, if $A = [a_{ij}]_{m \times n}$, then $A' = [a_{ji}]_{n \times m}$.

Properties of Transpose of a Matrix

For any matrices A and B of suitable orders:

(i) $(A')' = A$,

(ii) $(kA)' = kA'$ where k is a constant.

(iii) $(A + B)' = A' + B'$

(iv) $(AB)' = B' A'$

Symmetric and Skew Symmetric Matrix

If $A = [a_{ij}]$ be an $m \times n$ matrix,

(i) A is a symmetric matrix if $A' = A$

(ii) A is a skew symmetric matrix if A'= – A

Properties of Symmetric and Skew Symmetric Matrix

(i) For any square matrix A with real number elements, A + A' is a symmetric matrix and A – A' is a skew symmetric matrix.

(ii) Any square matrix can be represented as the sum of a symmetric and skew symmetric matrix.

(iii) If A and B are two symmetric or skew symmetric matrices of same order, then A + B also has the same order.

(iv) If A and B are two symmetric matrices of same order, then the product AB is symmetric if and only if AB = BA

Elementary Matrix

A matrix is called an elementary matrix if it can be obtained from identity matrix by performing a single row or column operation.

Row Transformations

(i) A row within the matrix can be interchanged with another row. $R_i \leftrightarrow R_j$

(ii) Each element in a row can be multiplied by a non zero constant. $R_i \rightarrow kR_i$ where $k \neq 0$.

(iii) A row can be replaced by the sum of that row and a multiple of another row. $R_i \rightarrow R_i + kR_j$ where k is a constant.

Column Transformations

(i) A column within the matrix can be interchanged with another column. $C_i \rightarrow C_j$

(ii) Each element in a column can be multiplied by a non zero constant. $C_i \rightarrow kC_i$ where $k \neq 0$.

(iii) A column can be replaced by the sum of that column and a multiple of another column. $C_i \rightarrow C_i + kC_j$ where k is a constant.

Invertible Matrix

If A and B are two square matrices such that AB = BA = I, then B is the inverse matrix of A denoted by A^{-1} and A is the inverse of B denoted by B^{-1}.

• A rectangular matrix does not posses an inverse.

• Inverse of a square matrix, if it exists, is unique.

• If A and B are invertible matrices of the same order, then $(AB)^{-1} = B^{-1}A^{-1}$

• $(A^{-1})^{-1} = A$

• $(kA)^{-1} = k^{-1}A^{-1}$ for non zero scalar k.

Inverse of a Matrix by Elementary Operations

Inverse by Elementary Row Operation

(i) If A is a matrix such that A^{-1} exists, then to find A^{-1} by elementary row operations, write A = IA

(ii) Apply a series of row operations on A = IA till I = BA is obtained.

(iii) The matrix B will be the inverse of A.

Inverse by Elementary Column Operation

(i) If A is a matrix such that A^{-1} _____ $^{-1}$ by elementary column operations, write A = AI.

(ii) Apply a series of column operations on A = AI till I = AB is obtained.

(iii) The matrix B will be the inverse of A.

Note:

If after applying one or more elementary row (or column) operations on A = IA (A = AI), we obtain all zeros in one or more rows of the matrix A on L.H.S., then A^{-1} does not exist.

DETERMINANT

If P is the set of square matrices, Q is the set of numbers (real or complex) and f _____ $f(A) = k$, where A ∈ P and k ∈ Q, then $f(A)$ is called the determinant of A. It is also denoted

If $A = \begin{bmatrix} a & b \\ c & d \end{bmatrix}$, then $\det(A) = |A| = \begin{bmatrix} a & b \\ c & d \end{bmatrix}$

Note: Determinants exist only for square matrices.

Determinant of a Matrix of Order 1

If A = [a] is a matrix of order 1, then det A = a

Determinant of a Matrix of Order 2

If $A = \begin{bmatrix} a & b \\ c & d \end{bmatrix}$ is a matrix of order 2 × 2,

then det (A) = |A| = $\begin{vmatrix} a & b \\ c & d \end{vmatrix}$ = $ad - bc$

Determinant of a Matrix of Order 3

If $A = \begin{bmatrix} a_1 & b_1 & c_1 \\ a_2 & b_2 & c_2 \\ a_3 & b_3 & c_3 \end{bmatrix}$ is a matrix of order 3 × 3, then

$|A| = \begin{vmatrix} a_1 & b_1 & c_1 \\ a_2 & b_2 & c_2 \\ a_3 & b_3 & c_3 \end{vmatrix} = a_1 \begin{vmatrix} b_2 & c_2 \\ b_3 & c_3 \end{vmatrix} - b_1 \begin{vmatrix} a_2 & c_2 \\ a_3 & c_3 \end{vmatrix} + c_1 \begin{vmatrix} a_2 & b_2 \\ a_3 & b_3 \end{vmatrix}$

Note: A determinant of a matrix of order 3 can be expanded in six ways (three along rows R_1, R_2, R_3 and three along column C_1, C_2, C_3).

Note:

- We expand the determinant along that row or column which contains maximum number of zeros.
- While expanding, we can multiply by $+1$ or -1 accordingly as $(i + j)$ is even or odd.
- If $A = kB$ where A and B are square matrices of order n, then $|A| = k^n |B|$ where $n = 1, 2, 3$

Properties of Determinant

(i) The value of a determinant remains unchanged if its rows and columns are interchanged.

If $R_i \leftrightarrow C_i$ where R_i is the ith row and C_i is the ith column, then $|A|$ does not change.

(ii) If any two rows or any two columns of a determinant are interchanged, then the sign of determinant changes.

If $R_i \leftrightarrow R_j$ or $C_i \leftrightarrow C_j$, then $|A| = - |A|$

(iii) If any two rows or any two columns of a determinant are identical, then the value of the determinant is zero.

If $R_i = R_j$ or $C_i = C_j$, then $|A| = 0$

(iv) If each element of a row or each element of a column of a determinant is multiplied by a constant k, then the value of the determinant gets multiplied by k.

If $R_i \rightarrow kR_i$ or $C_i \rightarrow kC_i$ where $k \neq 0$, then $|A| = k |A|$

(v) If some or all elements of a row or column of a determinant can be expressed as sum of two or more elements, then the determinant can be expressed as the sum of two or more determinants.

(vi) If to each element of any row or column of a determinant, the equimultiples of corresponding elements of other row or column are added, then the value of the determinant remains the same.

If $R_i \rightarrow R_i + kR_j$ or $C_i \rightarrow C_i + kC_j$, then $|A|$ does not change.

Area of a Triangle

The area of a triangle with vertices (x_1, y_1), (x_2, y_2) and (x_3, y_3) is given by

$$\text{Area of triangle} = \frac{1}{2} \begin{vmatrix} x_1 & y_1 & 1 \\ x_2 & y_2 & 1 \\ x_3 & y_3 & 1 \end{vmatrix}$$

(i) Since area is a positive quantity, we always take the absolute value of the determinant while calculating the area.

(ii) Use both positive and negative values of the determinant for calculation when the area is given.

(iii) The area of the triangle formed by three collinear points is zero.

Minor and Cofactor

Minor of an element a_{ij} of a determinant is the determinant obtained by deleting its ith row and j^{th} column in which element a_{ij} lies. Minor of an element a_{ij} is denoted by M_{ij}.

- Minor of an element of a determinant of order $n(n \geq 2)$ is a determinant of order $n - 1$.

Cofactor of an element a_{ij} of a determinant is defined by

$A_{ij} = (-1)^{i+j} M_{ij}$ where A_{ij} is the cofactor and M_{ij} is the minor of a_{ij}.

- If elements of a column are multiplied by the cofactors of any other column, then their sum is zero.
- If elements of a row are multiplied by the cofactors of any other row, then their sum is zero.

Adjoint of a Matrix

The adjoint of a square matrix $A = [a_{ij}]_{n \times n}$ is defined as the transpose of the matrix $[A_{ij}]_{n \times n}$, where A_{ij} is the cofactor of the element a_{ij}. Adjoint of the matrix A is represented by adjA.

If $A = \begin{vmatrix} a_{11} & a_{12} & a_{13} \\ a_{21} & a_{22} & a_{23} \\ a_{31} & a_{32} & a_{33} \end{vmatrix}$ then

$adj\ A = \text{Transpose of } \begin{vmatrix} A_{11} & A_{12} & A_{13} \\ A_{21} & A_{22} & A_{23} \\ A_{31} & A_{32} & A_{33} \end{vmatrix} = \begin{vmatrix} A_{11} & A_{21} & A_{31} \\ A_{12} & A_{22} & A_{32} \\ A_{13} & A_{23} & A_{33} \end{vmatrix}$

Property of Adjoint of a Matrix

If A be any given square matrix of order n, then

$A(adjA) = (adjA)\ A = |A|\ I$, where I is the identity matrix of order n.

Singular and Non Sigular Matrix

A square matrix A is said to be singular if $|A| = 0$

A square matrix A is said to be non singular if $|A| \neq 0$

Important Theorems

(i) If A and B are nonsingular matrices of the same order, then AB and BA are also nonsingular matrices of the same order.

(ii) The determinant of the product of matrices is equal to product of their respective determinants, $|AB| = |A|\ |B|$, where A and B are square matrices of the same order.

(iii) A square matrix A is invertible if and only if A is a non singular matrix.

Inverse of a Matrix

$$A^{-1} = \frac{1}{|A|} adj\, A$$

Consistent and Inconsistent System

Consistent : A system of equations is said to be consistent if there exists one or more solution.

Inconsistent : A system of equations is said to be inconsistent if there is no solution.

Application of Inverse of a Matrix

Let the system of equations be

$$a_1x + b_1y + c_1z = d_1$$
$$a_2x + b_2y + c_2z = d_2$$
$$a_3x + b_3y + c_3z = d_3$$

The given system of equations can be represented as AX = B or

$$\begin{bmatrix} a_1 & b_1 & c_1 \\ a_2 & b_2 & c_2 \\ a_3 & b_3 & c_3 \end{bmatrix} \begin{bmatrix} x \\ y \\ z \end{bmatrix} = \begin{bmatrix} d_1 \\ d_2 \\ d_3 \end{bmatrix} \text{ where } A = \begin{bmatrix} a_1 & b_1 & c_1 \\ a_2 & b_2 & c_2 \\ a_3 & b_3 & c_3 \end{bmatrix}, X = \begin{bmatrix} x \\ y \\ z \end{bmatrix} \text{ and } B = \begin{bmatrix} d_1 \\ d_2 \\ d_3 \end{bmatrix}$$

Case I

by $X = A^{-1}B$. This matrix equation gives a unique solution. This method is known as *Matrix Method* of solving a system of equations.

Case II

If A is a singular matrix, then $|A| = 0$. We calculate (adj A) B to solve the system of equations.

If (adj A) B = 0, then the system of equations may be either consistent

solution.

equations is called inconsistent.

LOGARITHM

Logarithm of a positive number x to the base a is the power of y to which the base must be raised in order to produce the number x.

If $\log_a x = y$, then $a^y = x$ where $a > 0$ and a

Properties of Logarithms

(i) $\log_a(xy) = \log_a x + \log_a y$

(ii) $\quad \log_a\left(\dfrac{x}{y}\right) = \log_a x - \log_a y$

(iii) $\quad \log_x x = 1$

(iv) $\quad \log_a 1 = 0$

(v) $\quad \log_a(x^n) = n(\log_a x)$

(vi) $\quad \log_a x = \dfrac{1}{\log_x a}$

(vii) $\quad \log_a x = \dfrac{\log_b x}{\log_b a} = \dfrac{\log x}{\log a}$

(viii) $\quad \log_b \sqrt[p]{x} = \dfrac{\log_b(x)}{p}$

Note:

$\quad log\ (a + b) \neq log\ a + log\ b$

$\quad log\ (a - b) \neq log\ a - log\ b$

$\quad$ If $y = log\ (a + b)$ it means $10^y = a + b$

$\quad$ Similarly, if $y = log\ (a - b)$ it means $10^y = a - b$

Change of base

The logarithm $log_b(x)$ can be calculated from the logarithms of x and b with respect to an arbitrary base k using the following formula:

$$\log_b(x) = \dfrac{\log_k(x)}{\log_k(b)}$$

Three commonly used bases of logarithm are binary logarithm (base 2), natural logarithm (base e) and common logarithm (base 10).

Logarithms with respect to any base b can be determined using either of these two logarithms by the previous formula:

$$\log_b(x) = \dfrac{\log_{10}(x)}{\log_{10}(b)} = \dfrac{\log_e(x)}{\log_e(b)}$$

Given a number x and its logarithm $log_b(x)$ to an unknown base b, the base is given by:

$$b = x^{\frac{1}{\log_b(x)}}$$

Common Logarithm

Logarithms to the base 10 are known as common logarithms.

Some frequently used common logarithms are:

$\log_{10} 10 = 1$

$\log_{10} 100 = 2$ since $10^2 = 100$

$\log_{10} 1000 = 3$ since $10^3 = 1000$

$\log_{10} 0.1 = -1$ since $10^{-1} = 0.1$

$\log_{10} 0.01 = -2$ since $10^{-2} = 0.01$

$\log_{10} 0.001 = -3$ since $10^{-3} = 0.001$

Characteristic and Mantissa

The logarithm of a number contains two parts, '**characteristic**' and '**mantissa**'.

Characteristic: The internal part of the logarithm of a number is called its *characteristic.*

Case I: When the number is greater than 1

In this case, the characteristic is one less than the number of digits in the left of the decimal point in the given number.

Case II: When the number is less than 1

In this case, the characteristic is one more than the number of zeros between the decimal point and the first significant digit of the number and it is negative.

Mantissa: The decimal part of the logarithm of a number is known as its *mantissa.* For mantissa, we look through log table.

Natural Logarithm

The natural logarithm of a number is its logarithm to the base e, where e is an irrational and transcendental constant approximately equal to 2.718281828. The natural logarithm of x is generally written as *ln x* or $log_e x$.

The natural logarithm function, if considered as a real-valued function of a real variable, is the inverse function of the exponential function.

$$e^{\ln(x)} = x$$
$$\text{if } x > 0$$
$$\ln(e^x) = x$$

All the properties of logarithm of general base is also true for common

Comparison of Properties of Common Logarithm, Natural Logarithm and General Logarithm

Common Logarithm Base 10	Natural Logarithm Base e	General Logarithm Base b
$\log x = y$ $10^y = x$	$\ln x = y$ $e^y = x$	$\log_b x = y$ $b^y = x$
$\log 1 = 0$	$\ln 1 = 0$	$\log_b 1 = 0$
$\log 10 = 1$	$\ln e = 1$	$\log_b b = 1$
$\log 10^x = x$ for all x	$\ln e^x = x$ for all x	$\log_b b^x = x$ for all x
$10^{\log x} = x,\ x > 0$	$e^{\ln x} = x,\ x > 0$	$b^{\log x} = x\ x > 0$
Product Property $\log AB = \log A + \log B$ and $\log A + \log B = \log AB$	Product Property $\ln AB = \ln A + \ln B$ and $\ln A + \ln B = \ln AB$	Product Property $\log_b AB = \log_b A + \log_b B$ and $\log_b A + \log_b B = \log_b AB$
Quotient Property $\log \dfrac{A}{B} = \log A - \log B$ and $\log A - \log B = \log \dfrac{A}{B}$	Quotient Property $\ln \dfrac{A}{B} = \ln A - \ln B$ and $\ln A - \ln B = \ln \dfrac{A}{B}$	Quotient Property $\log_b \dfrac{A}{B} = \log_b A - \log_b B$ and $\log_b A - \log_b B = \log_b \dfrac{A}{B}$
Power Property $\log B^t = t \log B$ and $t \log B = \log B^t$	Power Property $\ln B^t = t \ln B$ and $t \ln B = \ln B^t$	Power Property $\log_b B^t = t\log_b B$ and $t \log_b B = \log_b B^t$

MATHEMATICAL INDUCTION

Deduction is the application of a general case to a particular case.

Induction means generalization from a particular case.

Principle of Mathematical Induction

Let P(n) be a statement involving the natural number n such that

(i) The statement is true for $n = 1$, i.e., P(1) is true,

(ii) If the statement is true for $n = k$ (where k is some positive integer), then the statement is also true for $n = k + 1$, i.e., truth of $P(k)$ implies the truth of $P\ (k + 1)$.

Then, $P(n)$ is true for all natural numbers n.

EXPONENTIAL AND LOGARITHMIC SERIES

Series

If $a_1, a_2, a_3, ..., a_n$ be a given sequence,

then $a_1 + a_2 + a_3 + ... + a_n = \sum\limits_{k=1}^{n} a_k$ is known as a series associated with

the given sequence.

Finite Series

For example, $a + ar + ar^2 + ... + ar^{n-1}$

Infinite Series

series. For example, $a + ar + ar^2 + ... + ar^{n-1} + ...$

Sum of *n* Terms of Special Series

Sum of first *n* Natural Numbers

n natural numbers is given by

$$S_n = 1 + 2 + 3 + ... + n = \frac{n(n+1)}{2}$$

Sum of first *n* Odd Natural Numbers

n odd natural numbers is given by

$$S_n = 1 + 3 + ... + n = n^2$$

Sum of first *n* Even Natural Numbers

n even natural numbers is given by

$$S_n = 2 + 4 + ... + n = n(n+1)$$

Sum of Squares of first *n* Natural Numbers

n natural numbers is given by

$$S_n = 1^2 + 2^2 + 3^2 + ... + n^2 = \frac{n(n+1)(2n+1)}{6}$$

Sum of Squares of First *2n -1* Odd Natural Numbers

n- 1 odd natural numbers is given by

$$S_n = 1^2 + 3^2 + ... + (2n-1)^2 = \frac{n(2n-1)(2n+1)}{3}$$

Sum of Cubes of First *n* Natural Numbers

n natural numbers is given by

$$S_n = 1^3 + 2^3 + ... + n^3 = \frac{n^2(n+1)^2}{4} = \frac{[n(n+1)]^2}{4}$$

Exponential Series

$$e = 1 + \frac{1}{1!} + \frac{1}{2!} + \frac{1}{3!} + \frac{1}{4!} + \ldots$$

Also, $2 < e < 3$

The exponential series involving variable x is given by

$$e^x = \sum_{n=0}^{\infty} \frac{x^n}{n!} = 1 + x + \frac{x^2}{2!} + \frac{x^3}{3!} + \frac{x^4}{4!} + \ldots \quad -\infty < x < \infty$$

$$e^{-x^2} = 1 - x^2 + \frac{x^4}{2!} - \frac{x^6}{3!} + \frac{x^8}{4!} - \ldots -\infty < x < \infty$$

$$a^x = e^{x \ln \alpha} = 1 + \frac{x \ln a}{1!} + \frac{(x \ln a)^2}{2!} + \frac{(x \ln a)^3}{3!} + \ldots \quad -\infty < x < \infty$$

$$e^{\sin x} = 1 + x + \frac{x^2}{2} - \frac{x^4}{8} - \frac{x^5}{15} + \ldots \quad -\infty < x < \infty$$

$$e^{\cos x} = e\left(1 - \frac{x^2}{2} + \frac{x^4}{6} - \frac{31x^6}{720} + \ldots\right) \quad -\infty < x < \infty$$

$$e^{\tan x} = 1 + x + \frac{x^2}{2} + \frac{x^3}{2} + \frac{3x^4}{8} + \ldots \quad |x| < \frac{\pi}{2}$$

$$e^x \sin x = x + x^2 + \frac{x^3}{3} - \frac{x^5}{30} - \frac{x^6}{90} + \ldots + \frac{(\sqrt{2})^n \sin\left(\frac{n\pi}{4}\right) x^n}{n!} + \ldots \quad -\infty < x < \infty$$

$$e^x \cos x = 1 + x - \frac{x^3}{3} - \frac{x^4}{6} + \ldots + \frac{(\sqrt{2})^n \cos\left(\frac{n\pi}{4}\right) x^n}{n!} + \ldots \quad -\infty < x < \infty$$

Logarithmic Series

If $|x| < 1$ then,

$$\log_e (1 + x) = x - \frac{x^2}{2} + \frac{x^3}{3} - \ldots$$

The series on the right hand side of the above expansion is known as logarithmic series

For $x = 1$ we get, $\log_e 2 = 1 - \frac{1}{2} + \frac{1}{3} + \frac{1}{4} + \ldots$

Natural Logarithmic Series

$$\ln (1 + x) = \sum_{n=1}^{\infty} \frac{(-1)^{n+1}}{n} x^n = x - \frac{x^2}{2} + \frac{x^3}{3} - \ldots, \text{ for } -1 < x \leq 1$$

$$\ln (x) = (x - 1) - \frac{(x-1)^2}{2} + \frac{(x-1)^3}{3} - \frac{(x-1)^4}{4} \ldots, \text{ for } 0 < x \leq 2$$

3

Geometry Formulae

BASICS OF EUCLID'S GEOMETRY

Axiom and Theorem

The assumptions which are obvious universal truths are called *axioms*. They are not proved. The statements which are proved, using

theorems.

Euclid's Axioms

(i) *Transitive Property of Equality* : Things which are equal to the same thing are equal to one another.

(ii) *Addition Property of Equality* : If equals are added to equals, the wholes are equal.

(iii) *Subtraction Property of Equality* : If equals are subtracted from equals, the remainders are equal.

(iv)   : Things which coincide with one another are equal to one another.

(v) The whole is greater than the part.

Euclid's Postulates

Postulate 1 : A straight line segment can be drawn joining any two points.

Postulate 3 : A circle can be drawn with any given point as its centre and any distance as radius.

Postulate 4 : All right angles are congruent (equal to one another).

Postulate 5 : If a straight line falling on two straight lines makes the interior angles on the same side of it taken together less than two right

that side on which the sum of angles is less than two right angles.

(i) For every line *l* and for every point P not lying on *l*, there exists a unique line *m* passing through P and parallel to *l*.

(ii) Two distinct intersecting lines cannot be parallel to the same line.

LINE, LINE SEGMENT AND RAY

zero thickness.

A **line** is a group of points on a straight path that

Any two points on the line can be used to name it. This line is called line AB.

Line AB $(\overleftrightarrow{AB})$

A **line segment** is a part of a line that has two end points i.e. it has a starting point and an end

The two end points of the line segment are used to name the line segment. This line segment is called segment AB.

Line segment AB $(\overline{AB})$

A **ray** is a part of a line. It has one end point and

point on the ray.

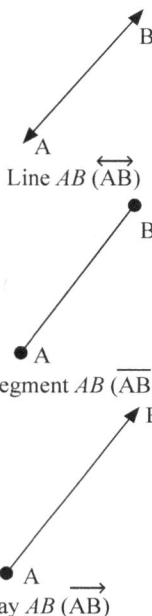

Ray AB $(\overrightarrow{AB})$

ANGLES

An angle is a measure of rotation of a given ray about its initial point. The initial point is known as the *vertex*. The initial ray is known as the *initial side*
terminal side of the angle.

If the direction of rotation is clockwise, then the angle is *negative* and if the direction of rotation is anticlockwise, the angle is said to be *positive*.

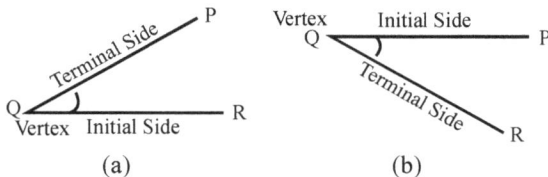

(a)   (b)

Unit of Angle
The unit of angle is degree or radian. The angle subtended at the centre by two unit radii and an arc of length 1 unit is known as 1 radian.

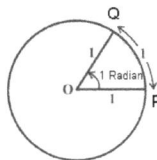

Relation between Degree and Radian

2π Radian $= 360°$

Or π Radian $= 180°$

Radian measure $= \dfrac{\pi}{180} \times$ Degree measure

Degree measure $= \dfrac{180}{\pi} \times$ Radian measure

1 radian $= 57° \ 17'$ approximately.

$1° = 0.017453$ radian approximately.

Acute Angle

An angle whose measure is between 0° and 90° is called an acute angle.

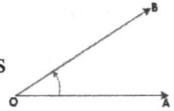

Right Angle

An angle whose measure is equal to 90° is called a right angle.

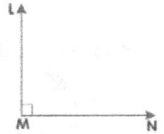

Obtuse Angle

An angle whose measure is greater than 90° but less than 180° is called an obtuse angle.

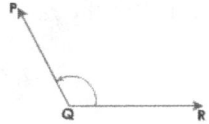

Straight Angle

An angle whose measure is equal to 180° is called a straight angle.

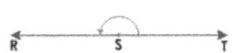

Reflex Angle

An angle whose measure is greater than 180° but less than 360° is called a reflex angle.

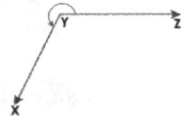

Complete Angle

One complete revolution from the position of the initial side is known as a complete angle. The measure of a complete angle is 360°

Adjacent Angles

Two angles are said to be adjacent if they have a common arm, a common vertex and are non overlapping.

$\angle$AOB and $\angle$BOC are adjacent angles. Here, OB is the common arm and O is the common vertex.

When two angles are adjacent, their sum is always equal to the angle formed by two non common arms.

$\angle$AOB $+ \angle$BOC $= \angle$AOC

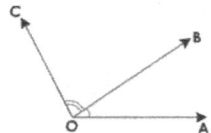

Complementary Angles

Two angles are said to be complementary angles, if the sum of their measures is equal to 90°. These may be adjacent angles as well.

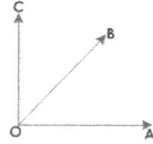

∠AOB and ∠BOC are adjacent angles as well as complementary angles.

∠AOB + ∠BOC = 90°

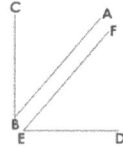

∠ABC and ∠DEF are complementary angles but not adjacent since they don't have a common arm or a common vertex.

∠ABC + ∠DEF = 90°

Supplementary Angles

Two angles are said to be supplementary if the sum of their measures is equal to 180°. These may be adjacent angles as well.

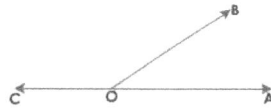

∠AOB and ∠BOC are supplementary as well as adjacent.

∠AOB + ∠BOC = 180°

∠ABC and ∠DEF are supplementary but not adjacent.

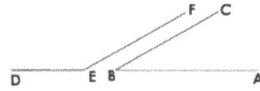

∠ABC + ∠DEF = 180°

Linear Pair

Two angles that are adjacent as well as supplementary are said to form a linear pair.

∠AOB and ∠ BOC form a linear pair.

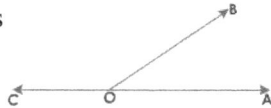

∠AOB + ∠ BOC = 180°

Vertically Opposite Angles

When two lines intersect the angles opposite to each other are known as vertically opposite angles. They are always equal.

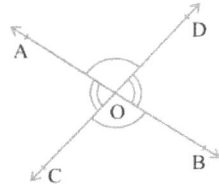

∠AOD and ∠ BOC, ∠AOC and ∠ BOD are vertically opposite angles.

∠AOD = ∠ BOC, and ∠ AOC = ∠ BOD

Some important Axioms

(i) If a ray stands on a line, then the sum of two adjacent angles so formed is 180°.

(ii) If the sum of two adjacent angles is 180°, then the non-common arms of the angles form a straight line.

PARALLEL AND PERPENDICULAR LINES

Lines are parallel if they lie in the same plane, and are the same distance apart over their entire length.

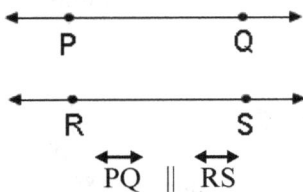

$$\overleftrightarrow{PQ} \parallel \overleftrightarrow{RS}$$

Two lines or line segments are said to be perpendicular if they are at right angles to each other.

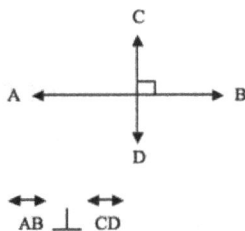

$$\overleftrightarrow{AB} \perp \overleftrightarrow{CD}$$

Intersecting Lines

Two or more lines that meet at a point are called intersecting lines.

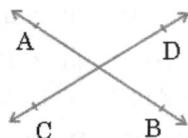

Note:

Two lines in a plane can either be parallel or intersecting.

Transversal

A line which intersects two or more lines at distinct points is known as a transversal.

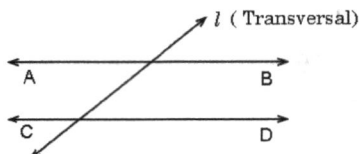

Angles formed by Parallel Lines

If two parallel lines are intersected by a transversal, then

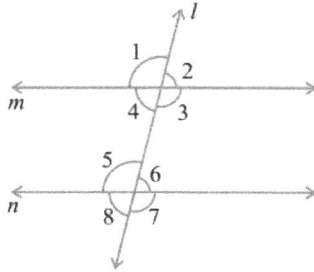

(i) Each pair of corresponding angles is equal.

$\angle 1 = \angle 5, \angle 2 = \angle 6, \angle 4 = \angle 8, \angle 3 = \angle 7$

(ii) Each pair of alternate interior angles is equal.

$\angle 4 = \angle 6, \angle 3 = \angle 5$

(iii) Each pair of alternate exterior angles is equal.

$\angle 1 = \angle 7, \angle 2 = \angle 8$

(iv) Each pair of interior angles on the same side of the transversal is supplementary.

$\angle 4 + \angle 5 = 180°$ and $\angle 3 + \angle 6 = 180°$

Converse Theorems

(i) If a transversal intersects two lines such that a pair of corresponding angles is equal, then the two lines are parallel to each other.

(ii) If a transversal intersects two lines such that a pair of alternate interior angles is equal, then the two lines are parallel.

(ii) If a transversal intersects two lines such that a pair of interior angles on the same side of the transversal is supplementary, then the two lines are parallel.

Lines Parallel to the Same Line

Lines which are parallel to the same line are parallel to each other.

$AB \parallel CD$ and $CD \parallel EF$ implies $AB \parallel EF$.

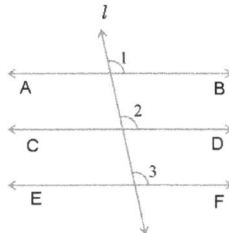

TRIANGLES

A triangle has six elements (three sides and three angles).

Scalene triangle: A scalene triangle is a triangle that has no equal sides.

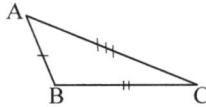

Isosceles triangle: An isosceles triangle is a triangle that has two equal sides.

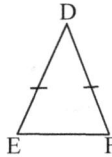

Equilateral triangle: An equilateral triangle is a triangle that has three equal sides.

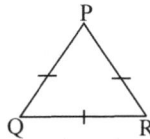

Right Angled Triangle
A right angled triangle is a triangle which has one right angle.

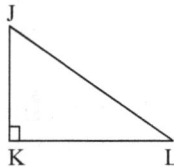

Obtuse Angled Triangle
An obtuse angled triangle is a triangle which has one obtuse angle.

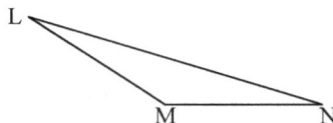

Mathematics Formulae

Acute Angled Triangle

An acute angled triangle is a triangle in which all the angles are less than 90 degrees, so all the angles are acute angles.

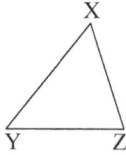

Naming Triangles Using Sides and Angles

- If a triangle has one right angle and two equal sides, we can call that triangle right isosceles triangle
- If a triangle has only acute angles and no equal sides, we can call that triangle acute scalene triangle.
- If a triangle has two equal sides and one obtuse angle, we can call that triangle obtuse isosceles triangle.

Note:

An equilateral triangle cannot have an obtuse angle or a right angle because all 3 angles in an equilateral triangle measure 60 degrees.

Exterior Angle of a Triangle

An exterior angle of a triangle is formed when a side of a triangle is produced. At each vertex, we have two ways of forming an exterior angle.

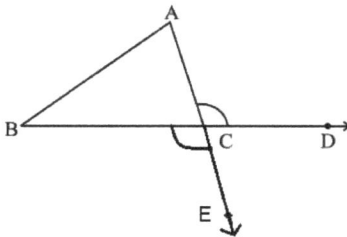

At vertex C, angle ACD and angle BCE are the two ways of forming an exterior angle.

Median, Altitude and Perpendicular bisector of a Triangle

Median of a triangle : A line segment joining the vertex of a triangle to the mid point of the opposite side is known as the median of a triangle. A triangle has 3 medians.

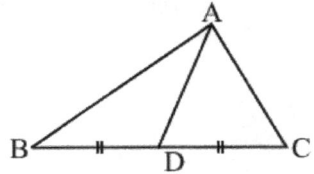

AD is the median of $\triangle$ABC.

Properties of Median

(i) Each median divides the triangle into two parts, and the areas of these two parts are equal.

In triangle ABC, the median AD divides the triangle into two parts: $\triangle$ADC and $\triangle$BDA.

Area of $\triangle$ADC = Area of $\triangle$BDA

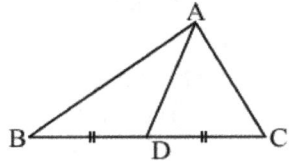

(ii) The three medians of a triangle are **concurrent.** i.e. they meet at a single point known as the **Centroid**. The medians AL, BM and CN meet at P, the centroid of the triangle.

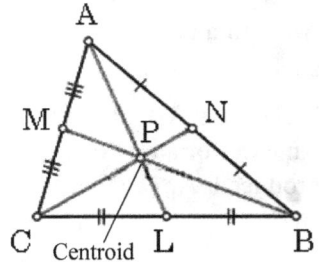

(iii)**Apollonius's Theorem** : The sum of the squares of any two sides of any triangle equals twice the square on half the third side, together with twice the square on the median bisecting the third side.

In any triangle ABC if AD is a median, then

$$AB^2 + AC^2 = 2(AD^2 + BD^2)$$

(iv) In $\triangle$ABC if a, b and c are the sides of the triangle with respective medians m_a, m_b, and m_c from their midpoints, then the lengths of the medians is given by:

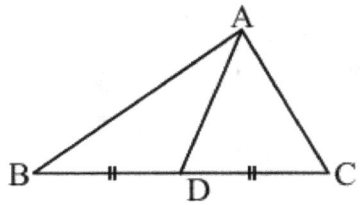

$$m_a = \sqrt{\frac{2b^2 + 2c^2 - a^2}{4}}$$

$$m_b = \sqrt{\frac{2a^2 + 2c^2 - b^2}{4}}$$

$$m_c = \sqrt{\frac{2a^2 + 2b^2 - c^2}{4}}$$

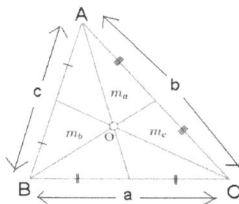

(v) Sum of the medians is less than the perimeter of the triangle.

$$m_a + m_b + m_c < AB + BC + CA$$

(vi) The medians from sides of lengths a and b are perpendicular if and only if:

$$a^2 + b^2 = 5c^2$$

(vii) Three times the sum of the square of the sides is equal to four times the sum of the square of the medians.

$$\frac{3}{4}(a^2 + b^2 + c^2) = m_a^2 + m_b^2 + m_c^2$$

(viii) The area of the triangle in terms of the median is given by:

$$\text{Area} = \frac{4}{3}\sqrt{s(s - m_a)(s - m_b)(s - m_c)}$$

$$\text{where } S = \frac{m_a + m_b + m_c}{2}$$

(ix) The centroid divides each median into two parts in the ratio 2:1, with the centroid being twice as close to the midpoint of a side as it is to the opposite vertex.

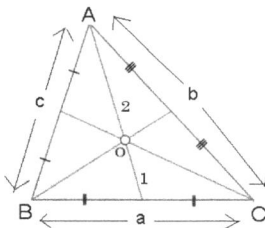

Altitude of a triangle : The perpendicular line segment from a vertex of a triangle to its opposite side is called an altitude of the triangle. A triangle has 3 altitudes.

PM is the altitude of $\triangle$PQR.

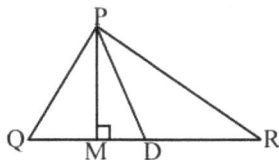

Properties of Altitude

(i) The point where all the altitudes of a triangle meet is known as the **orthocenter**. Altitudes AD, BE and CF meet at O the orthocenter of the triangle.

(ii) Orthocenter of a triangle is not always inside the triangle. It lies inside for an acute triangle, outside for an obtuse triangle and on the vertex of the right triangle.

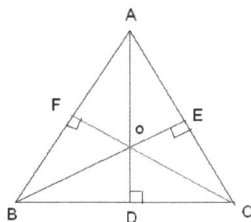

Orthocenter of Acute Triangle

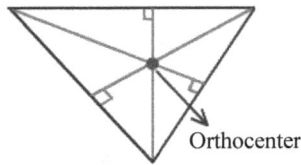

Orthocenter

Orthocenter of Right Triangle

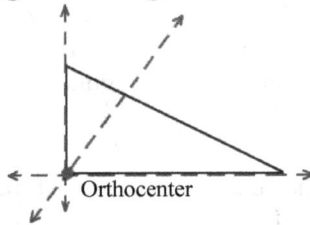

Orthocenter

Orthocenter of Obtuse Triangle

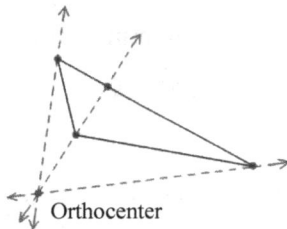

Orthocenter

Perpendicular Bisector of a Triangle

A line segment that is both perpendicular and passes through the mid point of a side of a triangle is called the perpendicular bisector of the triangle. A triangle has 3 perpendicular bisectors. It may or may not join the opposite vertex.

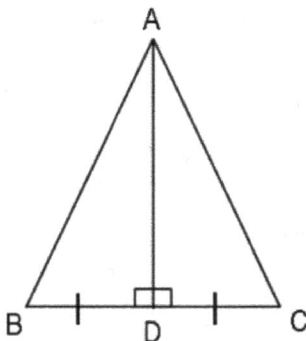

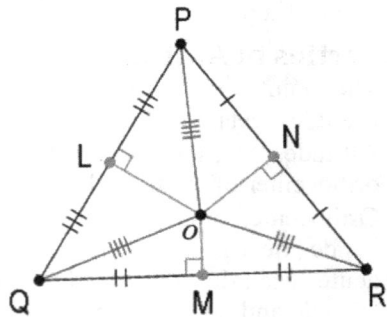

AD is the perpendicular bisector of ΔABC. OM, ON and OL are the perpendicular bisectors of ΔPQR.

Properties of Perpendicular Bisector

(i) The perpendicular bisectors of a triangle are concurrent. The point where three perpendicular bisectors of a triangle meet is known as the circumcenter.

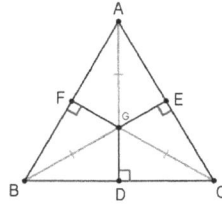

The perpendicular bisectors AD, BE and CF meet at a point G .

(ii) The circumcenter is equidistant from the vertices of the triangle i.e. GA = GB = GC

(iii) The circle that passes through all the three vertices of the triangle is known as circumcircle of a triangle. The circumcenter is the centre of the circumcircle.

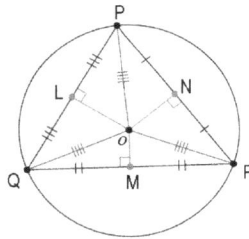

O is the centre of the circumcircle. OP, OQ and OR are the circumradius of the circumcircle.

a) Every triangle has a circumcircle.

b) The position of the circumcenter depends on the type of the triangle. It lies inside an acute triangle, outside an obtuse triangle and at the centre of the hypotenuse on a right triangle.

Note:

- In case of an equilateral triangle the centroid, incenter and circumcenter are coincident.
- Every perpendicular bisector is an altitude but every altitude is not a perpendicular bisector.
- Every perpendicular bisector is a median but every median is not a perpendicular bisector.

Angle Bisector of a Triangle

Definition

An angle bisector is a line segment or ray that divides an angle into two congruent angles.

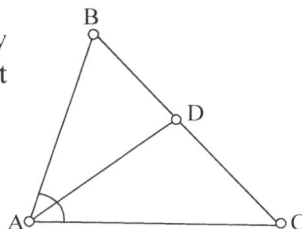

AD is the angle bisector of ∠ BAC i.e.

∠ BAD = ∠ DAC

Properties of Angle Bisector of a Triangle

(i) If a point lies on the bisector of an angle, then it is equidistant from the sides of the angle.

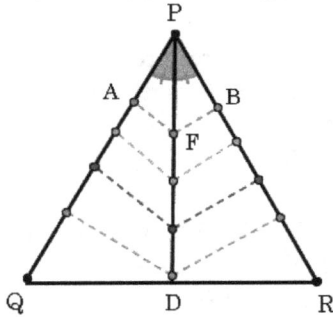

If PD is the angle bisector of $\angle$QPR, then AF = BF

(ii) *Angle Bisector Theorem* : This theorem states that the angle bisector of a triangle divides the sides of the triangle proportionally.

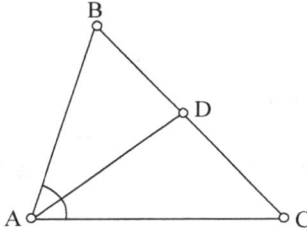

In $\triangle$ABC, if AD is the bisector of $\angle$BAC, then

$$\frac{BD}{DC} = \frac{AB}{AC}$$

(iii) The three angle bisectors of a triangle are concurrent. The point where the three angle bisectors of a triangle meet is called the incenter. The circle drawn with centre at incentre and radius equal to the perpendicular distance from incentre to any side of a triangle is known as incircle.

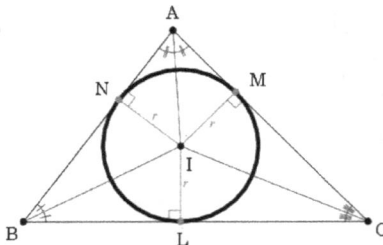

Mathematics Formulae

IL, IM and IN are the inradius.

CONGRUENCE OF TRIANGLES

Two triangles are congruent, if their corresponding sides are equal in length and their corresponding angles are equal in size. If triangle ABC is congruent to triangle DEF, the relationship can be written mathematically as:

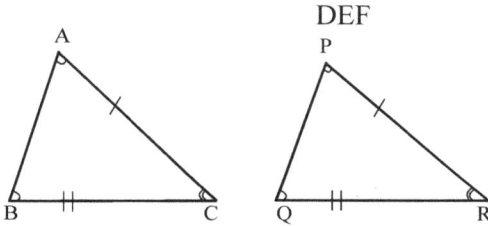

(i)   Corresponding vertices: A and P, B and Q, C and R.
(ii) Corresponding sides: AB and PQ, BC and QR, AC and PR .
(iii) Corresponding angles: A and   P,   B and   Q,   C and   R.

Properties of Congruence of Triangles
Reflexive Property
Every triangle is congruent to itself.
Symmetric Property
ABC

Transitive Property

PQR.

Congruency Rules
Side Side Side (SSS)
If three sides of one triangle are equal to the corresponding three sides of the other triangle, then the two triangles are congruent.

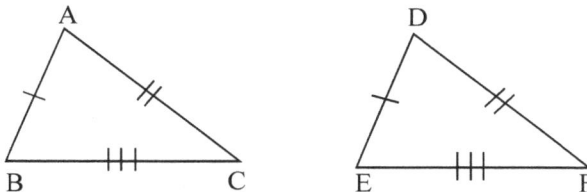

Side Angle Side (SAS)

If two sides and the included angle of one triangle are equal to two sides and the included angle of the other triangle, then the two triangles are congruent.

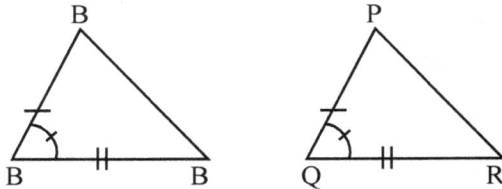

In $\triangle ABC$ and $\triangle PQR$, $AB = QP$, $AC = QR$ and $\angle BAC = \angle PQR$, hence $\triangle ABC \cong \triangle QPR$ by SAS congruency rule.

Angle Side Angle (ASA)

If two angles and the included side of one triangle are equal to two angles and the included side of the other triangle, then the two triangles are congruent.

In $\triangle DEF$ and $\triangle PQR$, $EF = QR$, $\angle DEF = \angle PQR$ and $\angle DFE = \angle PRQ$, hence $\triangle DEF \cong \triangle PQR$ by ASA congruency rule.

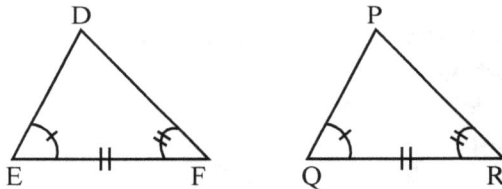

Angle Angle Side (AAS)

If two angles and one side of one triangle are equal to two angles and the corresponding side of the other triangle, then the two triangles are congruent.

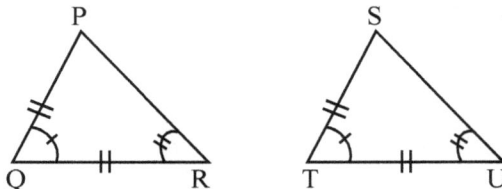

In $\triangle PQR$ and $\triangle STU$, $PQ = ST$, $\angle PQR = \angle STU$ and $\angle QRP = \angle TUS$, hence $\triangle PQR \cong \triangle STU$ by AAS congruency rule.

RHS Rule

If in two right triangles, hypotenuse and one side of a triangle are equal to the hypotenuse and one side of other triangle, then the two triangles are congruent.

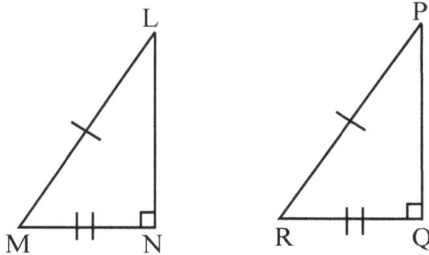

In $\triangle$LMN and $\triangle$PRQ, LM = PR, MN = RQ and
$\angle$LNM = $\angle$PQR = 90°, then $\triangle$LNM $\cong$ $\triangle$PQR by RHS congruency rule.

Properties of a Triangle

(i) Exterior Angle Property

The measure of any exterior angle of a triangle is equal to the sum of the measures of its interior opposite angles.

$$\angle 1 + \angle 2 = \angle ACD$$

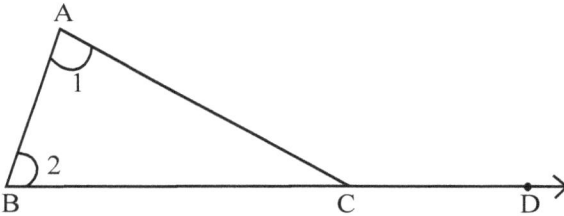

(ii) Angle Sum Property of a Triangle

The sum of the measure of three angles of a triangle is 180°.

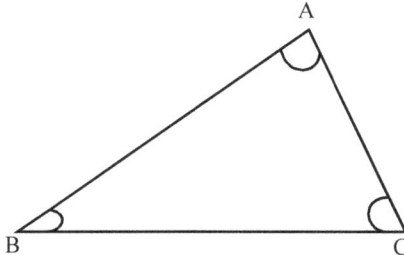

$$\angle A + \angle B + \angle C = 180°$$

(iii)Angles opposite to equal sides of a triangle are equal.

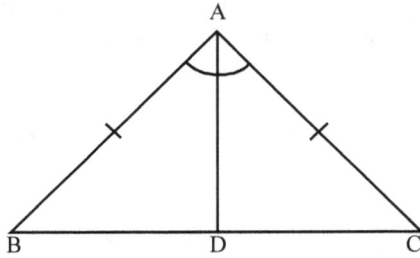

If AB = AC, ∠ACB = ∠ABC

(iv)Sides opposite to equal angles of a triangle are equal.

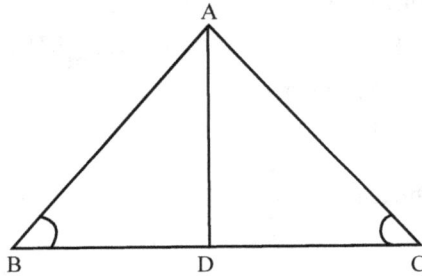

If ∠ACB = ∠ABC, then AB = AC

(v) Each angle of an equilateral triangle is of 60°.

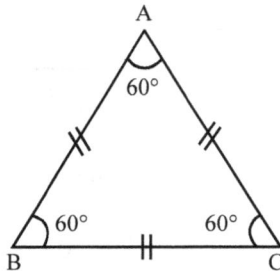

(vi)In a triangle, angle opposite to the longer side is larger (greater). In ΔABC, AC is the largest side, hence, ∠ABC is the largest angle.

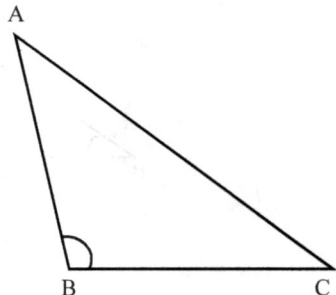

(vii) In a triangle, the side opposite to the larger (greater) angle is longer.

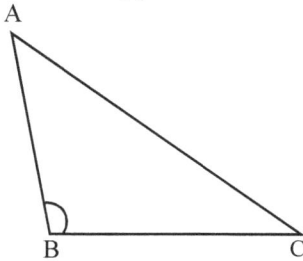

In $\triangle ABC$, $\angle ABC$ is the largest angle, hence AC is the largest side.

(viii) Sum of any two sides of a triangle is greater than the third side

$$AB + AC > BC$$
$$AB + BC > AC$$
$$BC + AC > AB$$

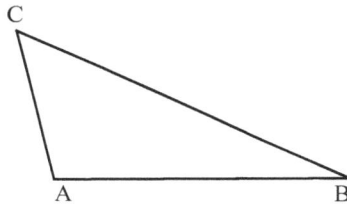

(ix) Two triangles on the same base (or equal bases) and between the same parallels are equal in area.

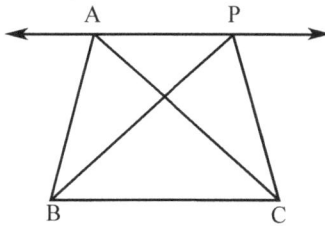

$\triangle ABC$ and $\triangle PBC$ lie on the same base BC and lie between the same parallels BC and AP hence, $ar(\triangle ABC) = ar(\triangle PBC)$.

(x) Two triangles having equal areas and the same base (or equal bases) lie between the same parallels.

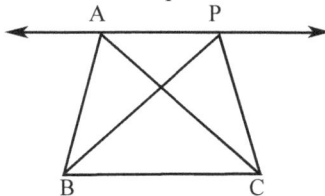

$ar(\triangle ABC) = ar(\triangle PBC)$ and they lie on the same base BC, hence they lie between same parallels AP and BC.

Mid Point Theorem

The line segment joining the mid-points of two sides of a triangle is parallel to the third side and half of it.

If E and F are the mid points of sides

then

$$EF \parallel BC \text{ and } EF = \frac{1}{2}BC$$

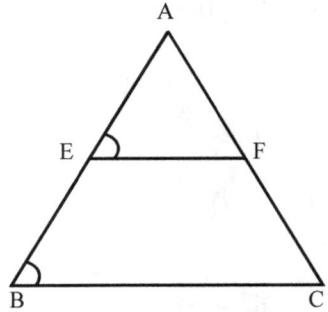

Converse of Mid Point Theorem

The line drawn through the mid-point of one side of a triangle, parallel to another side bisects the third side.

If E is the mid point of side AB of

point of side AC.

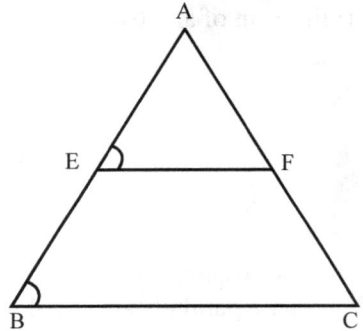

SIMILARITY OF TRIANGLES

Two triangles are similar, if
  (i) their corresponding angles are equal and
  (ii) their corresponding sides are in the same ratio (or proportion).

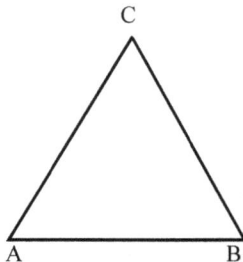

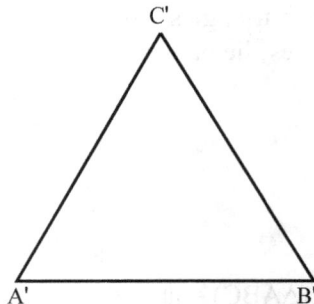

In $\triangle ABC$ and $\triangle A'B'C'$,

(i) $\angle A = \angle A'$, $\angle B = \angle B'$, $\angle C = \angle C'$

(ii) $\dfrac{AB}{A'B'} = \dfrac{BC}{B'C'} = \dfrac{CA}{C'A'}$

Hence, $\triangle ABC \sim \triangle A'B'C'$

Note: All congruent triangles are similar but all similar triangles are not congruent.

If corresponding angles of two triangles are equal, then they are known as **equiangular triangles**.

The ratio of any two corresponding sides in two equiangular triangles is always the same.

Similarity Criterion

AAA similarity : If in two triangles, corresponding angles are equal, then their corresponding sides are in the same ratio and hence the two triangles are similar by AAA similarity criterion.

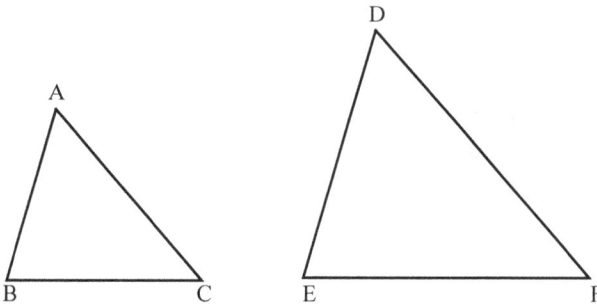

In $\triangle ABC$ and $\triangle DEF$,

if $\angle A = \angle D$, $\angle B = \angle E$ and $\angle C = \angle F$

then $\dfrac{AB}{DE} = \dfrac{BC}{EF} = \dfrac{CA}{DF}$

$\triangle ABC \sim \triangle DEF$ (AAA Similarity)

AA similarity : If in two triangles, two angles of one triangle are respectively equal to the two angles of the other triangle, then the two triangles are similar by AA similarity criterion.

If two angles of a triangle are respectively equal to two angles of another triangle, then by the angle sum property of a triangle their third angles will also be equal. Hence, AA similarity is same as AAA similarity.

SSS similarity : If in two triangles, corresponding sides are in the same ratio, then their corresponding angles are equal and hence the triangles are similar by SSS similarity criterion.

In $\triangle ABC$ and $\triangle DEF$,

if $\dfrac{AB}{DE} = \dfrac{BC}{EF} = \dfrac{AC}{DF}$

then $\angle A = \angle D$, $\angle B = \angle E$ and $\angle C = \angle F$

$\triangle ABC \sim \triangle DEF$ (SSS Similarity)

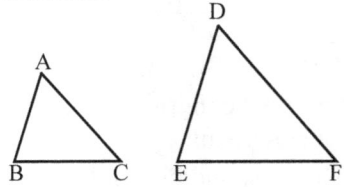

SAS similarity : If one angle of a triangle is equal to one angle of another triangle and the sides including these angles are in the same ratio (proportional), then the triangles are similar by SAS similarity criterion.

In $\triangle ABC$ and $\triangle DEF$,

if $\dfrac{AB}{DE} = \dfrac{AC}{DF}$ (<1) and $\angle A = \angle D$ then

$\triangle ABC \sim \triangle DEF$ (SAS Similarity)

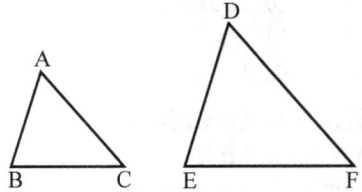

Properties of Similar Triangle

(i) **Basic Proportionality Theorem (Thales Theorem)** : If a line is drawn parallel to one side of a triangle to intersect the other two sides at distinct points, then the other two sides are divided in the same ratio.

In $\triangle ABC$, DE is parallel to BC and intersects AB at D and AC at E then

$$\frac{AD}{DB} = \frac{AE}{EC}$$

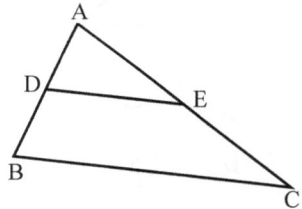

(ii) If a line divides any two sides of a triangle in the same ratio, then the line is parallel to the third side.

In $\triangle ABC$ if $\dfrac{AD}{DB} = \dfrac{AE}{EC}$

then DE $\parallel$ BC

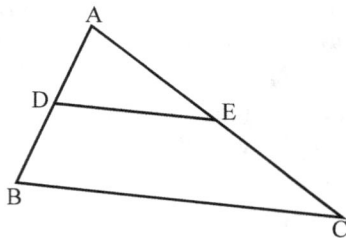

(iii) The ratio of the areas of two similar triangles is equal to the square of the ratio of their corresponding sides.

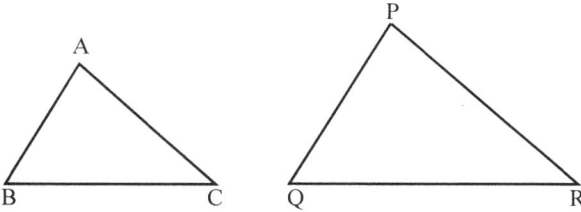

If $\triangle ABC \sim \triangle PQR$

then $\dfrac{ar(ABC)}{ar(PQR)} = \left(\dfrac{AB}{PQ}\right)^2 = \left(\dfrac{BC}{QR}\right)^2 = \left(\dfrac{CA}{RP}\right)^2$

(iv) Perimeters of similar triangles are in the same ratio as the scale factor (When two triangles are similar, the reduced ratio of any two corresponding sides is called the scale factor of the similar triangles).

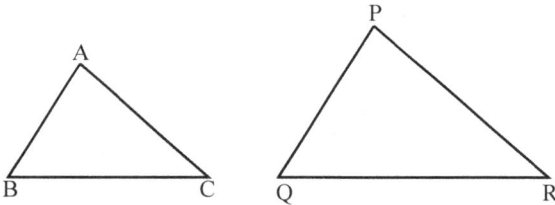

If $\triangle ABC \sim \triangle PQR$, then

$$\dfrac{\text{Perimeters of } \triangle ABC}{\text{Perimeters of } \triangle PQR} = \dfrac{\text{Length of AB}}{\text{Length of PQ}} = \dfrac{\text{Length of BC}}{\text{Length of QR}} = \dfrac{\text{Length of CA}}{\text{Length of RP}}$$

(v) If a perpendicular is drawn from the vertex of the right angle of a right triangle to the hypotenuse, then the triangles on both sides of the perpendicular are similar to the whole triangle and also to each other.

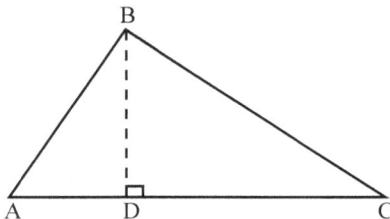

In right angled triangle ABC right angled at B, a perpendicular BD is drawn on the hypotenuse AC, then

QUADRILATERAL

A quadrilateral is a polygon with four sides and four vertices.

Quadrilateral	Properties
Square	
Rhombus	
Rectangle	
Parallelogram	
Trapezium	
Kite	is equal. other.

Note:

Every rectangle is a parallelogram but not vice versa.

Every square is a rhombus but not vice versa.

Some other Properties

- The sum of four interior angles of a quadrilateral is 360°.
- The quadrilateral formed by joining the mid-points of the sides of a quadrilateral, in order, is a parallelogram.

Condition for Quadrilateral to be a Parallelogram

A quadrilateral is a parallelogram, if

(i) opposite sides are equal or

(ii) opposite angles are equal or

(iii) a pair of opposite sides is equal and parallel or

(iv) diagonals bisect each other

Property of a Parallelogram

(i) Parallelograms on the same base and between the same parallels are equal in area.

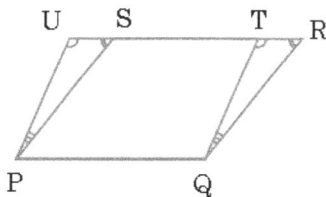

Parallelograms PQRS and PQTU are on the same base PQ and between same parallels PQ and UR, hence

$$ar(PQRS) = ar(PQTU)$$

(ii) Parallelograms on the same base (or equal bases) and having equal areas lie between the same parallels.

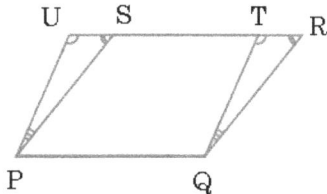

Parallelograms PQRS and PQTU are on the same base PQ and if ar(PQRS) = ar(PQTU), then the parallelograms lie between the same parallels PQ and UR.

Triangle and Parallelogram on the Same Base

If a triangle and a parallelogram are on the same base and between the same parallels, the area of the triangle is equal to half the area of the parallelogram.

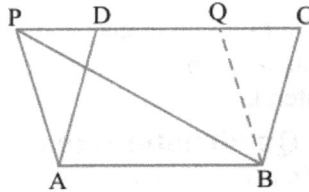

same parallels AB and PC then

$$\frac{1}{2} \text{ar(ABCD)}$$

CIRCLE

A circle is the collection of all points in a plane, which are equidistant **centre**

radius.

A line segment whose end points lie on the circle is known as a **chord**.

A chord which passes through the centre of the circle is known as a **diameter**. Diameter = 2 × Radius

Note:

Diameter is the longest chord of a circle.

Every diameter is a chord but every chord is not a diameter.

Circle and its Related Terms

Circular Region : A circle divides the plane on which it lies into three parts.

(i) Interior of the circle (inside portion of the circle)

(ii) The circle

(iii) Exterior of the circle (outside portion of the circle)

The circle along with its interior is called the circular region.

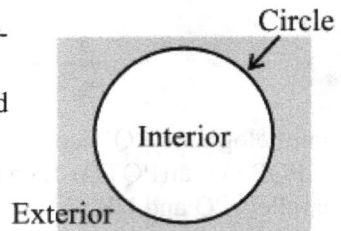

Mathematics Formulae

Circumference : The linear distance around the edge of a circle is known as circumference.

Arc : Any part of the circumference of a circle is known as an arc.

Major and Minor Arc : The larger arc joining two points on the circumference of a circle is known as a major arc. The shorter arc joining two points on the circumference of a circle is known as a minor arc.

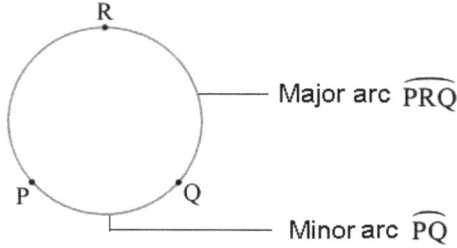

Major arc $\overgroup{PRQ}$

Minor arc $\overgroup{PQ}$

Segment of a Circle : The region between a chord and a major or minor arc is called a segment of a circle. The region between a chord and a major arc is called a *major segment* of a circle. The region between a chord and a *minor arc* is called a minor segment of a circle.

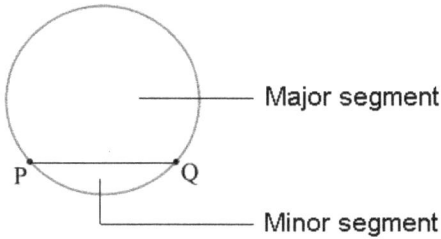

Major segment

Minor segment

Sector : The region between two radii and the arc joining the end points of the radii is known as a sector. The region between two radii and the minor arc is known as *minor sector*. The region between two radii and the major arc is known as *major sector*.

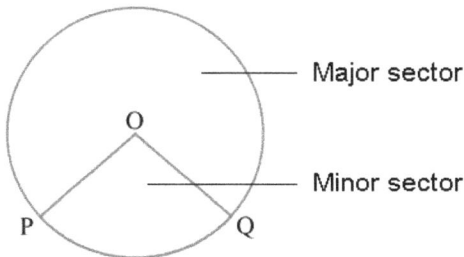

Major sector

Minor sector

Semi Circle : Half of a circle is known as a semi circle.

In a semi circle, the major arc is equal to the minor arc, the major segment is equal to the minor segment and the major sector is equal to the minor sector.

Cyclic Quadrilateral

A quadrilateral ABCD is said to be cyclic if all the four vertices A, B, C and D lie on the circle.

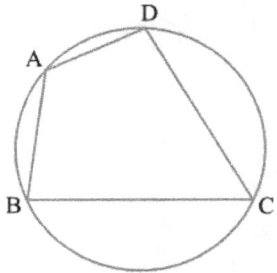

Tangent of a Circle

A line that intersects the circle at only one point is known as the tangent of a circle.

- The common point of the tangent and the circle is called the point of contact and the tangent is said to touch the circle at the point of contact.
- There is only one tangent at a point of the circle.
- The line containing the radius through the point of contact is called the normal to the circle at the point.

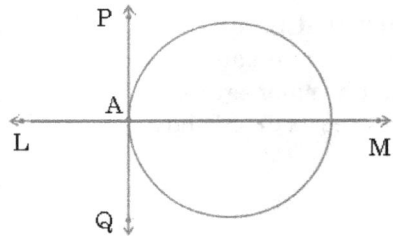

Line PQ is the tangent of the circle. Point A is the point of contact. Line LM is the normal.

Length of Tangent

Length of the tangent from an external point is the length of the segment between the external point and the point of contact.

PQ and PR are the length of the tangents from an external point P of the circle.

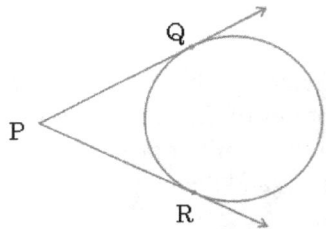

Secant of a Circle

A line that intersects the circle at two points is known as the secant of a circle.

- The tangent to a circle is a special case of the secant, when the two end points of its corresponding chord coincide.

Line PQ is the secant of the circle.

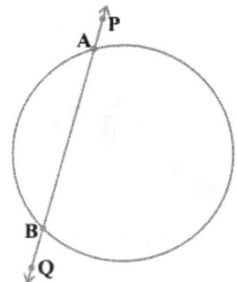

Properties of a Circle

(i) Equal chords of a circle (or of congruent circles) subtend equal angles at the centre.

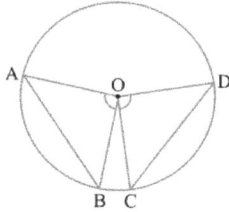

If chord AB is equal to chord CD of a circle with centre O, then
$\angle AOB = \angle COD$

(ii) If the angles subtended by two chords of a circle (or of congruent circles) at the centre (corresponding centres) are equal, the chords are equal.

If $\angle AOB = \angle COD$ in a circle with centre O, then chord AB = chord CD.

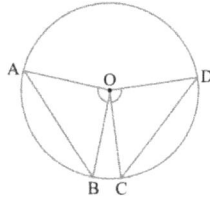

(iii) The perpendicular from the centre of a circle to a chord bisects the chord.

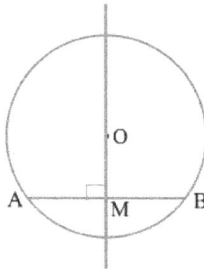

If $\angle OMA = \angle OMB = 90°$ in a circle with centre O and chord AB, then AM = MB.

(iv) The line drawn through the centre of a circle to bisect a chord is perpendicular to the chord.

If OM is drawn in such a way that
AM = MB, then $\angle OMB = 90°$

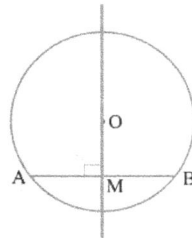

(v) There is one and only one circle passing through three non-collinear points.

There is only one circle passing through three non collinear points A, B and C.

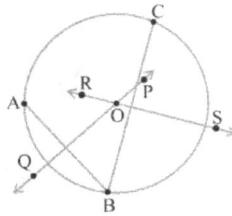

(vi) Equal chords of a circle (or of congruent circles) are equidistant from the centre (or corresponding centres).

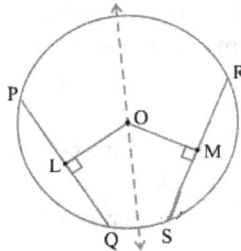

If chord PQ is equal to chord RS, then the perpendicular distance from the centre, OL = OM.

(vii) Chords equidistant from the centre (or corresponding centres) of a circle (or of congruent circles) are equal.

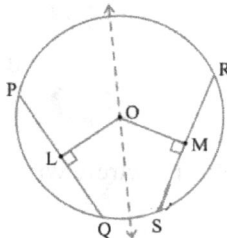

If the perpendicular distance from the centre OL = OM, then the chord PQ = chord RS.

(viii) If two arcs of a circle are congruent, then their corresponding chords are equal and conversely. If two chords of a circle are equal, then their corresponding arcs (minor, major) are congruent.

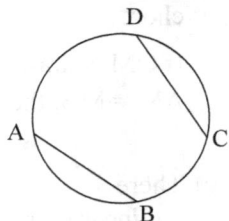

If chord AB = chord DC, then arc AB = arc DC and if arc AB = arc DC, then chord AB = chord DC.

(ix) Congruent arcs of a circle subtend equal angles at the centre.

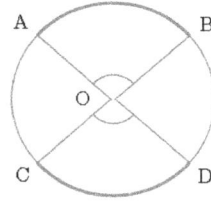

If arc AB = arc CD, then ∠AOB = ∠COD

(x) The angle subtended by an arc at the centre is double the angle subtended by it at any point on the remaining part of the circle.

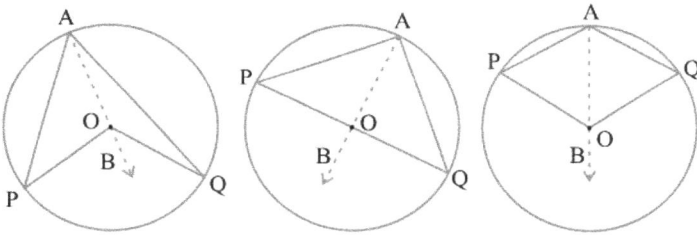

If arc PQ of the circle subtends an angle POQ at the centre and PAQ at a point on the remaining part of the circle, then
$$\angle POQ = 2\angle PAQ$$

(xi) Angles in the same segment of a circle are equal.

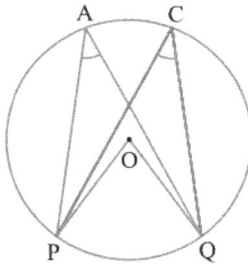

If two angles PCQ and PAQ are formed in the same segment, then
$$\angle PCQ = \angle PAQ$$

(xii) Angle in a semicircle is a right angle. If arc PAQ forms a semi circle, then
$$\angle PAQ = 90°$$

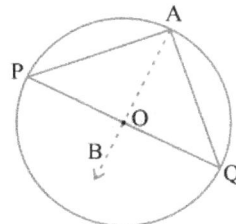

(xiii) If a line segment joining two points subtends equal angles at two other points lying on the same side of the line containing the line segment, the four points lie on a circle.

If a line segment AB subtends two equal angles ACB and ADB and if E and E' lie on the same side of AB as C and D, then E and E' coincide with D.

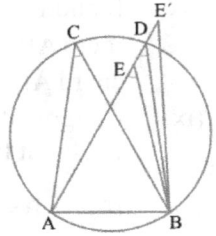

(xiv) The sum of either pair of opposite angles of a cyclic quadrilateral is 180^0.
If ABCD is a cyclic quadrilateral, then
$\angle A + \angle C = \angle B + \angle D = 180°$

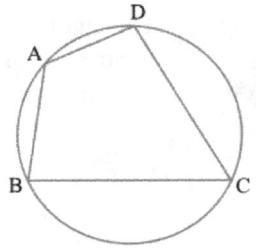

(xv) If sum of a pair of opposite angles of a quadrilateral is 180^0, the quadrilateral is cyclic.

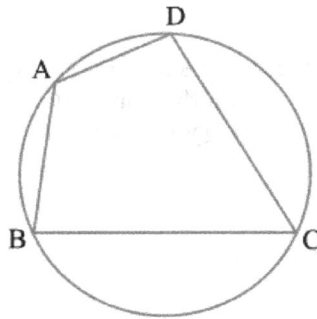

If $\angle A + \angle C = \angle B + \angle D = 180°$, then quadrilateral ABCD is a cyclic quadrilateral.

Properties of a Tangent

(i) The tangent to a circle is perpendicular to the radius through the point of contact.

If XY is a tangent to the circle with point of contact P, then the radius OP is perpendicular to the tangent at P.

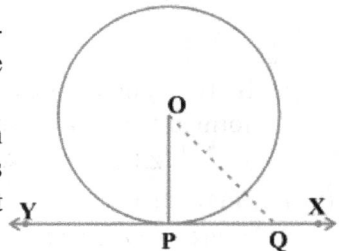

Mathematics Formulae

(ii) The lengths of the two tangents from an external point to a circle are equal.

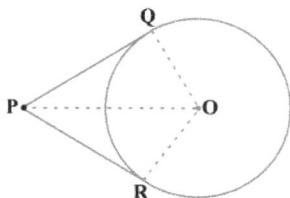

If a point P lies outside a circle with centre O and two tangents PQ and PR are drawn, then PQ = PR.

POLYGON

Types of Polygon

(i) **Regular Polygon**: A regular polygon has sides of equal length and all its interior angles are of equal measure. Regular polygons are both equiangular and equilateral.

(ii) **Irregular Polygon**: Irregular polygons can have sides of any length and angles of any measure.

Polygons of all types can be regular or irregular.

Name	Regular	Irregular
Triangle		
Quadrilateral		
Pentagon		
Hexagon		
Octagon		

(iii) **Equiangular Polygon** : In this polygon, all angles are equal.

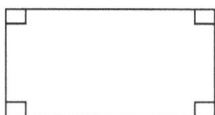

Rectangle

(iv) **Equilateral Polygon** : In this polygon, all sides are equal.

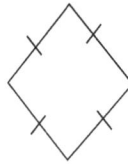

Rhombus

(v) **Convex Polygon** : A polygon with all its interior angles less than or equal to 180° is known as a convex polygon. In a convex polygon, every line segment between two vertices remains inside or on the boundary of the polygon. The Regular polygons are always convex.

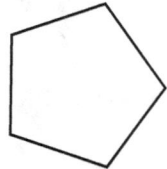

Regular Pentagon

(vi) **Concave Polygon** : A polygon with one or more interior angles greater than 180^0 is known as a concave polygon.

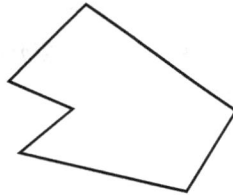

(vii) **Crossed Polygon** : A polygon where one or more sides crossed back over itself is called a crossed polygon. Most of the properties and theorems concerning polygons do not apply to this shape.

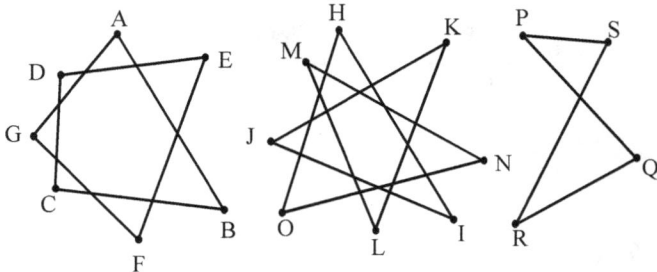

Similarity of Polygons

Two polygons of the same number of sides are similar, if

(i) their corresponding angles are equal and

(ii) their corresponding sides are in the same ratio (or proportion).

Properties of Polygons (Regular and Irregular)

(i) **Interior angles** : For a regular polygon all the interior angles are the same. For an irregular polygon, each angle may be different.

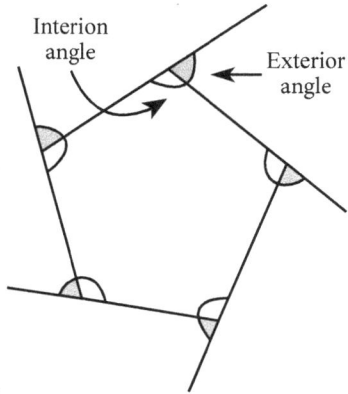

Interion angle

Exterior angle

a) The sum of the interior angles of a simple n-gon is $(n-2)\,\pi$ radians

or $(n-2)\,180°$, where n is the number of sides in a polygon.

b) Each interior angle is given by
$$\frac{(n-2)180°}{n}$$

(ii) a) The sum of the measures of the exterior angles of a polygon, one at each vertex is 360°.

b) Each angle of a regular convex polygon of n sides is $\dfrac{360}{n}$

3. **Diagonals** : The diagonals of a polygon are lines joining any two non-adjacent vertices. A diagonal may lie outside the polygon as well.

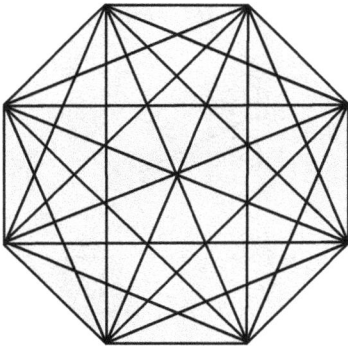

An octagon has
20 diagonals

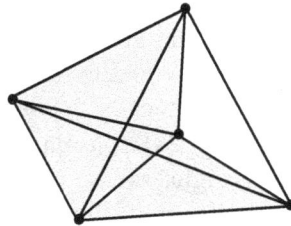

The number of diagonals of a n sided polygon is given by $\dfrac{n(n-3)}{2}$

4

Trigonometry Formulae

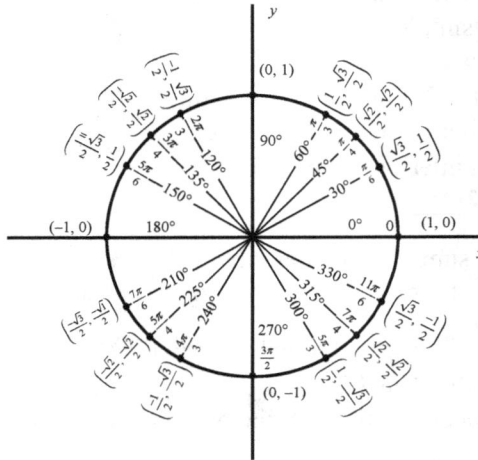

Cosine and Sine Around the Unit Circle

Pythagoras Theorem

In a right triangle, the square of the hypotenuse (the side opposite to the right angle) is equal to the sum of the square of the other two sides.

Converse of Pythagoras Theorem : If in a triangle, square of one side is equal to the sum of the squares of the

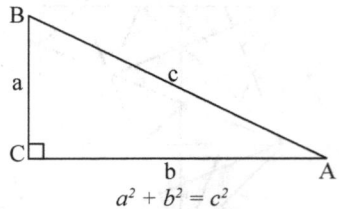

$$a^2 + b^2 = c^2$$

$^2 = a^2 + b^2$, then the angle opposite to side c i.e angle C is a right angle.

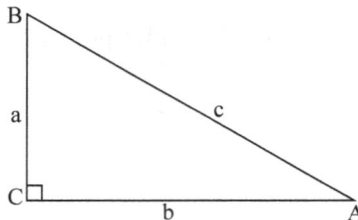

Pythagorean Triplet

For any natural number $n > 1$, $(2n)^2 + (n^2 - 1)^2 = (n^2 + 1)^2$. Hence $2n$, $n^2 - 1$ and $n^2 + 1$ form a Pythagorean triplet.

Trigonometric Ratio Definition

Trigonometric ratio is a ratio that describes a relationship between a side and angle of a right triangle.

Trigonometric Ratios in Right Triangles

There are six trigonometric ratios in right triangles.

$$\sin\theta = \frac{\text{length of opposite side}}{\text{length of hypotenuse}}$$

$$\cos\theta = \frac{\text{length of adjacent side}}{\text{length of hypotenuse}}$$

$$\tan\theta = \frac{\text{length of opposite side}}{\text{length of adjacent side}}$$

$$\sec\theta = \frac{\text{length of hypotenuse}}{\text{length of adjacent side}}$$

$$\mathrm{cosec}\,\theta = \frac{\text{length of hypotenuse}}{\text{length of opposite side}}$$

$$\cot\theta = \frac{\text{length of adjacent side}}{\text{length of opposite side}}$$

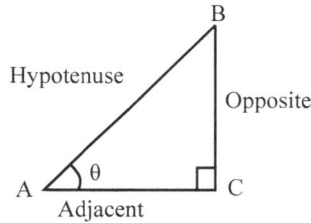

Relation Between Various Trigonometric Ratios

$$\tan\theta = \frac{\sin\theta}{\cos\theta}, \quad \sec\theta = \frac{1}{\cos\theta}$$

$$\mathrm{cosec}\,\theta = \frac{1}{\sin\theta}, \quad \cot\theta = \frac{1}{\tan\theta} = \frac{\cos\theta}{\sin\theta}$$

In terms of	$\sin \theta$	$\cos \theta$	$\tan \theta$	$\csc \theta$	$\sec \theta$	$\cot \theta$
$\sin \theta =$	$\sin \theta$	$\pm\sqrt{1-\cos^2\theta}$	$\pm\dfrac{\tan\theta}{\sqrt{1+\tan^2\theta}}$	$\dfrac{1}{\csc\theta}$	$\pm\dfrac{\sqrt{\sec^2\theta-1}}{\sec\theta}$	$\pm\dfrac{1}{\sqrt{1+\cot^2\theta}}$
$\cos \theta =$	$\pm\sqrt{1-\sin^2\theta}$	$\cos \theta$	$\pm\dfrac{1}{\sqrt{1+\tan^2\theta}}$	$\pm\dfrac{\sqrt{\csc^2\theta-1}}{\csc\theta}$	$\dfrac{1}{\sec\theta}$	$\pm\dfrac{\cot\theta}{\sqrt{1+\cot^2\theta}}$
$\tan \theta =$	$\pm\dfrac{\sin\theta}{\sqrt{1-\sin^2\theta}}$	$\pm\dfrac{\sqrt{1-\cos^2\theta}}{\cos\theta}$	$\tan \theta$	$\pm\dfrac{1}{\sqrt{\csc^2\theta-1}}$	$\pm\sqrt{\sec^2\theta-1}$	$\dfrac{1}{\cot\theta}$
$\csc \theta =$	$\dfrac{1}{\sin\theta}$	$\pm\dfrac{1}{\sqrt{1-\cos^2\theta}}$	$\pm\dfrac{\sqrt{1+\tan^2\theta}}{\tan\theta}$	$\csc \theta$	$\pm\dfrac{\sec\theta}{\sqrt{\sec^2\theta-1}}$	$\pm\sqrt{1+\cot^2\theta}$
$\sec \theta =$	$\pm\dfrac{1}{\sqrt{1-\sin^2\theta}}$	$\dfrac{1}{\cos\theta}$	$\pm\sqrt{1+\tan^2\theta}$	$\pm\dfrac{\csc\theta}{\sqrt{\csc^2\theta-1}}$	$\sec \theta$	$\pm\dfrac{\sqrt{1+\cot^2\theta}}{\cot\theta}$
$\cot \theta =$	$\pm\dfrac{\sqrt{1-\sin^2\theta}}{\sin\theta}$	$\pm\dfrac{\cos\theta}{\sqrt{1-\cos^2\theta}}$	$\dfrac{1}{\tan\theta}$	$\pm\sqrt{\csc^2\theta-1}$	$\pm\dfrac{1}{\sqrt{\sec^2\theta-1}}$	$\cot \theta$

Each trigonometric function in terms of the other five

Note: The values of the trigonometric ratios of an angle do not vary with the lengths of the sides of the triangle, if the angle remains the same.

Trigonometric Table

1 full circle = 360 degrees = 2π radians

θ (Radian)	0	$\dfrac{\pi}{6}$	$\dfrac{\pi}{4}$	$\dfrac{\pi}{3}$	$\dfrac{\pi}{2}$
θ (Degree)	$0°$	$30°$	$45°$	$60°$	$90°$
$\sin\theta$	0	$\dfrac{1}{2}$	$\dfrac{1}{\sqrt{2}}$	$\dfrac{\sqrt{3}}{2}$	1
$\cos\theta$	1	$\dfrac{\sqrt{3}}{2}$	$\dfrac{1}{\sqrt{2}}$	$\dfrac{1}{2}$	0
$\tan\theta$	0	$\dfrac{1}{\sqrt{3}}$	1	$\sqrt{3}$	Not defined
$\cot\theta$	Not defined	$\sqrt{3}$	1	$\dfrac{1}{\sqrt{3}}$	0
$\sec\theta$	1	$\dfrac{2}{\sqrt{3}}$	$\sqrt{2}$	2	Not defined
$\mathrm{cosec}\theta$	Not defined	2	$\sqrt{2}$	$\dfrac{2}{\sqrt{3}}$	1

Pythagorean Identity

$\sin^2\theta + \cos^2\theta = 1$, where $0° \leq \theta \leq 90°$

$1 + \tan^2\theta = \sec^2\theta$, where $0° \leq \theta < 90°$

$1 + \cot^2\theta = \operatorname{cosec}^2\theta$, where $0° < \theta \leq 90°$

Symmetry in Trigonometric Functions

$\sin(-\theta) = -\sin\theta$ $\cos(-\theta) = +\cos\theta$

$\tan(-\theta) = -\tan\theta$ $\csc(-\theta) = -\csc\theta$

$\sec(-\theta) = +\sec\theta$ $\cot(-\theta) = -\cot\theta$

Trigonometric Ratios of Complementary Angles

$\sin(\frac{\pi}{2} - \theta) = +\cos\theta$ $\cos(\frac{\pi}{2} - \theta) = +\sin\theta$

$\tan(\frac{\pi}{2} - \theta) = +\cot\theta$ $\csc(\frac{\pi}{2} - \theta) = +\sec\theta$

$\sec(\frac{\pi}{2} - \theta) = +\csc\theta$ $\cot(\frac{\pi}{2} - \theta) = +\tan\theta$

PERIODICITY IN TRIGONOMETRIC FUNCTIONS

$\sin(\theta + \frac{\pi}{2}) = +\cos\theta$ $\cos(\theta + \frac{\pi}{2}) = -\sin\theta$

$\tan(\theta + \frac{\pi}{2}) = -\cot\theta$ $\csc(\theta + \frac{\pi}{2}) = +\sec\theta$

$\sec(\theta + \frac{\pi}{2}) = -\csc\theta$ $\cot(\theta + \frac{\pi}{2}) = -\tan\theta$

$\sin(\theta + \pi) = -\sin\theta$ $\cos(\theta + \pi) = -\cos\theta$

$\tan(\theta + \pi) = +\tan\theta$ $\csc(\theta + \pi) = -\csc\theta$

$\sec(\theta + \pi) = -\sec\theta$ $\cot(\theta + \pi) = +\cot\theta$

$\sin(\pi - \theta) = +\sin\theta$ $\cos(\pi - \theta) = -\cos\theta$

$\tan(\pi - \theta) = -\tan\theta$ $\csc(\pi - \theta) = +\csc\theta$

$\sec(\pi - \theta) = -\sec\theta$ $\cot(\pi - \theta) = -\cot\theta$

$\sin(\theta + 2\pi) = +\sin\theta$ $\cos(\theta + 2\pi) = +\cos\theta$

$\tan(\theta + 2\pi) = +\tan\theta$ $\csc(\theta + 2\pi) = +\csc\theta$

$\sec(\theta + 2\pi) = +\sec\theta$ $\cot(\theta + 2\pi) = +\cot\theta$

$\sin(2\pi - \theta) = -\sin\theta$ $\cos(2\pi - \theta) = +\cos\theta$

$\tan(2\pi - \theta) = -\tan\theta$ $\csc(2\pi - \theta) = -\csc\theta$

$\sec(2\pi - \theta) = +\sec\theta$ $\cot(2\pi - \theta) = -\cot\theta$

Trigonometric Equations

$\sin\theta = 0$ implies $\theta = n\pi$, where n is any integer

$\cos\theta = 0$ implies $\theta = (2n + 1)\frac{\pi}{2}$ where n is any integer

$\sin x = \sin y$ implies $x = n\pi + (-1)^n y$, where $n \in Z$

$\cos x = \cos y$ implies $x = 2n\pi \pm y$, where $n \in Z$

$\tan x = \tan y$ implies $x = n\pi + y$, where $n \in Z$

Signs of Trigonometric Functions in Different Quadrants

	I	II	III	IV
Sinθ	+	+	−	−
Cosθ	+	−	−	+
Tanθ	+	−	+	−
Cosecθ	+	+	−	−
Secθ	+	−	−	+
Cotθ	+	−	+	−

Domain and Range of Trigonometric Functions

Trigono-metric Function	Domain	Range
$y = \sin x$	{Real numbers}	$[-1,1]$
$y = \cos x$	{Real numbers}	$[-1,1]$
$y = \tan x$	$\{x : x \in R \text{ and } x \neq (2n+1)\,\frac{\pi}{2}, n \in Z\}$	{Real numbers}
$y = \csc x$	$\{x : x \in R \text{ and } x \neq n\pi, n \in Z\}$	$\{y:y \in R, y \geq 1$ or $y \leq -1\}$
$y = \sec x$	$\{x : x \in R \text{ and } x \neq (2n+1)\,\frac{\pi}{2}, n \in Z\}$	$\{y:y \in R, y \geq 1$ or $y \leq -1\}$
$y = \cot x$	$\{x : x \in R \text{ and } x \neq n\pi, n \in Z\}$	{Real numbers}

Area of Triangle

If a, b, c are the lengths of sides of a triangle and A, B, C are the opposite angles, then

Area of $\triangle ABC = \dfrac{1}{2}ab\,\mathrm{Sin}\,C$

Or

Area of $\triangle ABC = \dfrac{1}{2}bc\,\mathrm{Sin}\,A$

Or

Area of $\triangle ABC = \dfrac{1}{2}ac\,\mathrm{Sin}\,B$

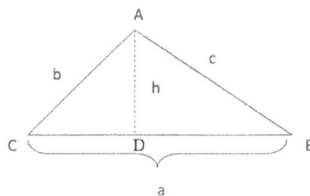

Law of Sine

If *a, b, c* are the lengths of sides of a triangle; A, B, C are the opposite angles and D is the diameter of the circumcircle of the triangle, then

$$\frac{a}{\sin A} = \frac{b}{\sin B} = \frac{c}{\sin C} = D$$

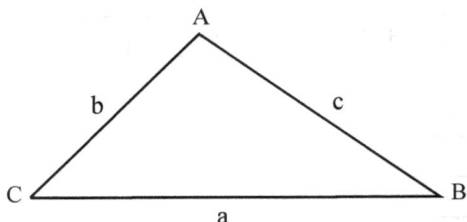

Law of Cosine

If *a, b, c* are the lengths of sides of a triangle; A, B, C are the opposite angles, then

$$c^2 = a^2 + b^2 - 2ab\,\cos C$$
$$a^2 = b^2 + c^2 - 2bc\,\cos A$$
$$b^2 = a^2 + c^2 - 2ac\,\cos B$$

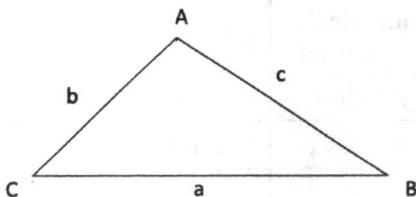

Double Angle

$$\sin(2A) = 2\sin(A)\cos(A)$$
$$\sin(2A) = \frac{2\tan(A)}{1+\tan^2(A)}$$
$$\cos(2A) = 1 - 2\sin^2(A)$$
$$\cos(2A) = 2\cos^2(A) - 1$$
$$\cos(2A) = \cos^2(A) - \sin^2(A)$$
$$\cos(2A) = \frac{1-\tan^2(A)}{1+\tan^2(A)}$$
$$\tan(2A) = \frac{2\tan(A)}{1-\tan^2(A)}$$

Half Angle

$$\sin\left(\frac{A}{2}\right) = \pm\sqrt{\frac{1-\cos(A)}{2}}$$

$$\cos\left(\frac{A}{2}\right) = \pm\sqrt{\frac{1+\cos(A)}{2}}$$

$$\tan\left(\frac{A}{2}\right) = \pm\frac{1-\cos(A)}{\sin(A)}$$

Triple Angle

$\sin(3A) = 3\sin(A) - 4\sin^3(A)$

$\cos(3A) = 4\cos^3(A) - 3\cos(A)$

$$\tan(3A) = \frac{3\tan(A) - \tan^3(A)}{1 - 3\tan^2(A)}$$

Sum to Product

$$\sin(A) + \sin(B) = 2\sin\left(\frac{A+B}{2}\right)\cos\left(\frac{A-B}{2}\right)$$

$$\sin(A) - \sin(B) = 2\cos\left(\frac{A+B}{2}\right)\sin\left(\frac{A-B}{2}\right)$$

$$\cos(A) + \cos(B) = 2\cos\left(\frac{A+B}{2}\right)\cos\left(\frac{A-B}{2}\right)$$

$$\cos(A) - \cos(B) = -2\sin\left(\frac{A+B}{2}\right)\sin\left(\frac{A-B}{2}\right)$$

Product to Sum

$2\cos(A)\cos(B) = \cos(A+B) + \cos(A-B)$

$-2\sin(A)\sin(B) = \cos(A+B) - \cos(A-B)$

$2\sin(A)\cos(B) = \sin(A+B) + \sin(A-B)$

$2\cos(A)\sin(B) = \sin(A+B) - \sin(A-B)$

Sum and Difference

$\sin(A + B) = \sin(A)\cos(B) + \cos(A)\sin(B)$

$\sin(A - B) = \sin(A)\cos(B) - \cos(A)\sin(B)$

$\cos(A + B) = \cos(A)\cos(B) - \sin(A)\sin(B)$

$\cos(A - B) = \cos(A)\cos(B) + \sin(A)\sin(B)$

$$\tan(A + B) = \frac{\tan(A) + \tan(B)}{1 - \tan(A)\tan(B)}$$

$$\tan(A - B) = \frac{\tan(A) - \tan(B)}{1 + \tan(A)\tan(B)}$$

$$\cot(A + B) = \frac{\cot(A)\cot(B) - 1}{\cot(B) + \cot(A)}$$

$$\cot(A - B) = \frac{\cot(A)\cot(B) + 1}{\cot(B) - \cot(A)}$$

Sum of Sine and Cosine

$$a_1\sin(Bt) + a_2\cos(Bt) = a\sin(Bt + \phi)$$

where $a = \sqrt{a_1 + a_2}$ and $\tan(\phi) = \dfrac{a_2}{a_1}$

ϕ satisfies $\cos(\phi) = \dfrac{a_1}{a}$ and $\sin(\phi) = \dfrac{a_2}{a}$

Euler's Formula

$e^{ix} = \cos x + i\sin x$, where $i = \sqrt{-1}$

$e^{i\pi} + 1 = 0$

Inverse Trigonometric Functions

The domain and range (principal value branch) of inverse trigonometric functions are given by:

Functions	Domain	Range (Principal Value Branch)
$y = \sin^{-1}x$	$[-1, 1]$	$\left[\dfrac{-\pi}{2}, \dfrac{\pi}{2}\right]$
$y = \cos^{-1}x$	$[-1, 1]$	$[0, \pi]$
$y = \csc^{-1}x$	$R - (-1, 1)$	$\left[\dfrac{-\pi}{2}, \dfrac{\pi}{2}\right] - \{0\}$
$y = \sec^{-1}x$	$R - (-1, 1)$	$[0, \pi] - \left\{\dfrac{\pi}{2}\right\}$
$y = \tan^{-1}x$	R	$\left(\dfrac{-\pi}{2}, \dfrac{\pi}{2}\right)$
$y = \cot^{-1}x$	R	$(0, \pi)$

Note:

$\sin^{-1}x \neq (\sin x)^{-1}$

$(\sin x)^{-1} = \dfrac{1}{\sin x}$

The other five trigononometric functions are also defined in a similar manner.

The value of an inverse trigonometric function which lies in its principal value branch is called the principal value of that inverse trigonometric function.

Whenever no branch of an inverse trigonometric function is mentioned, we mean the principal value branch of that function.

For suitable values of domain,

- $y = \sin^{-1}x \Rightarrow x = \sin y$
- $x = \sin y \Rightarrow y = \sin^{-1}x$
- $\sin(\sin^{-1}x) = x$
- $\sin^{-1}(\sin x) = x$
- $\sin^{-1}\dfrac{1}{x} = \cosce^{-1}x$
- $\cos^{-1}\dfrac{1}{x} = \sec^{-1}x$
- $\tan^{-1}\dfrac{1}{x} = \cot^{-1}x$
- $\sin^{-1}(-x) = -\sin^{-1}x$
- $\tan^{-1}(-x) = -\tan^{-1}x$
- $\cosec^{-1}(-x) = -\cosec^{-1}x$
- $\cos^{-1}(-x) = \pi - \cos^{-1}x$
- $\cot^{-1}(-x) = \pi - \cot^{-1}x$
- $\sec^{-1}(-x) = \pi - \sec^{-1}x$
- $\sin^{-1}x + \cos^{-1}x = \dfrac{\pi}{2}$
- $\tan^{-1}x + \cot^{-1}x = \dfrac{\pi}{2}$
- $\cosec^{-1}x + \sec^{-1}x = -$
- $\tan^{-1}x + \tan^{-1}y = \tan^{-1}\dfrac{x+y}{1-xy}$
- $\tan^{-1}x - \tan^{-1}y = \tan^{-1}\dfrac{x-y}{1+xy}$
- $2\tan^{-1}x = \tan^{-1}\dfrac{2x}{1-x^2}$
- $2\tan^{-1}x = \sin^{-1}\dfrac{2x}{1+x^2} = \cos^{-1}\dfrac{1-x^2}{1+x^2}$

Graph of Trigonometric Functions

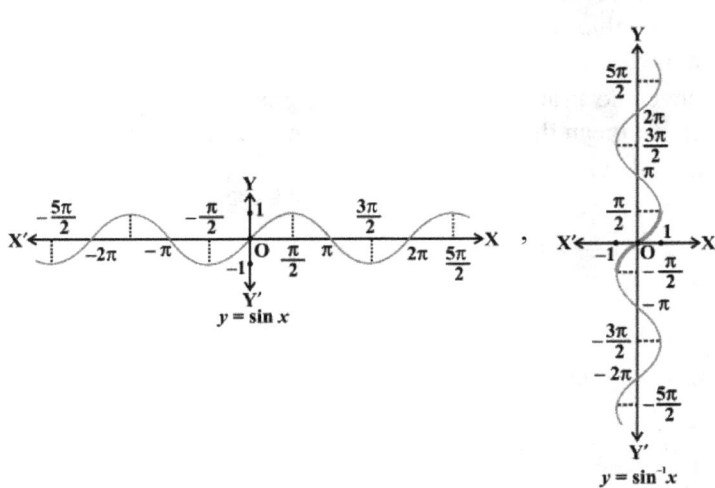

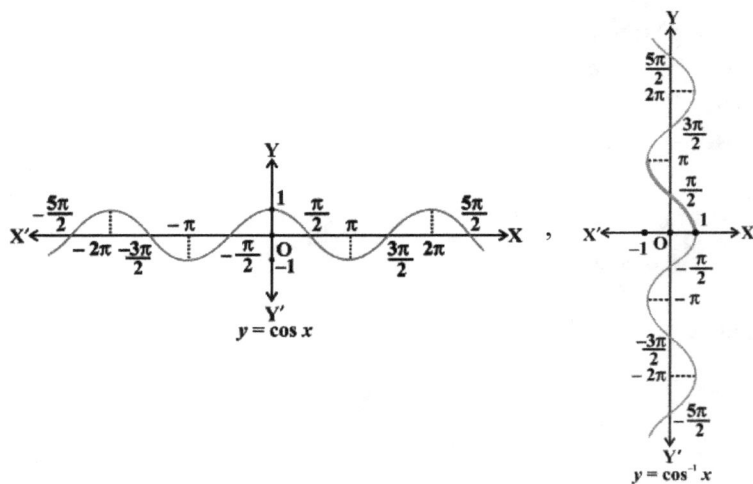

$y = \sin x$

$y = \sin^{-1} x$

$y = \cos x$

$y = \cos^{-1} x$

Mathematics Formulae

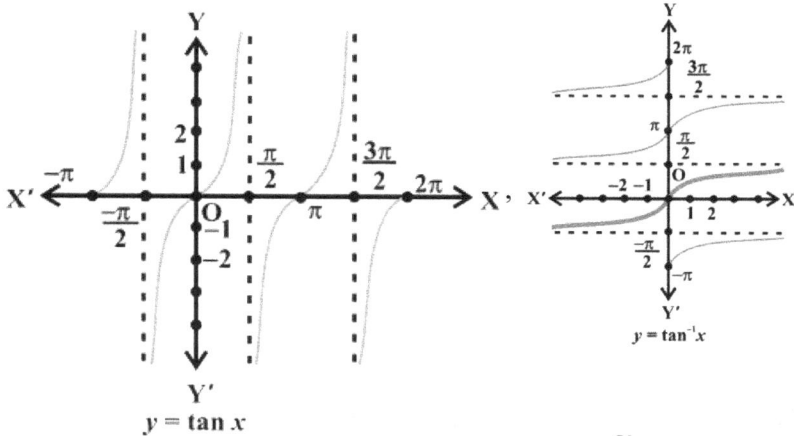

$y = \tan x$

$y = \tan^{-1} x$

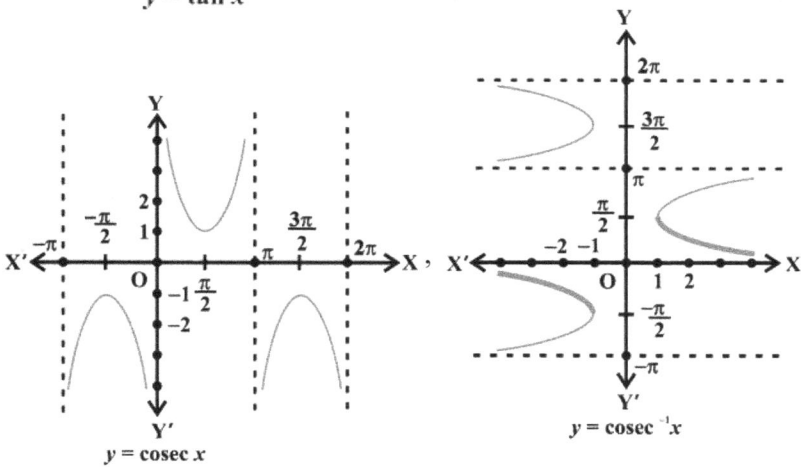

$y = \mathrm{cosec}\, x$

$y = \mathrm{cosec}^{-1} x$

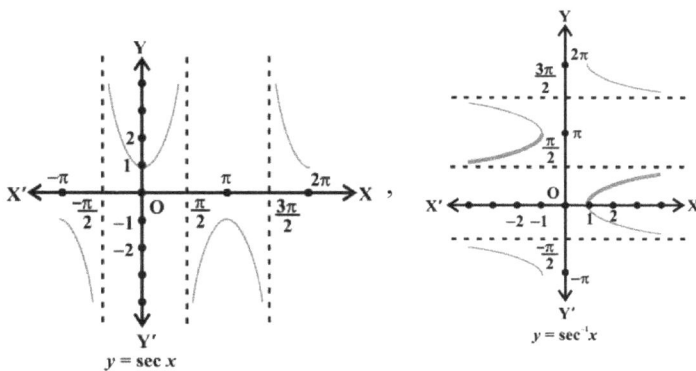

$y = \sec x$

$y = \sec^{-1} x$

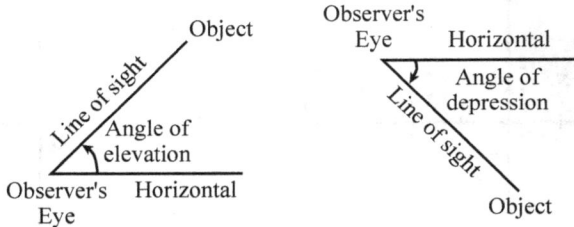

$y = \cot x$

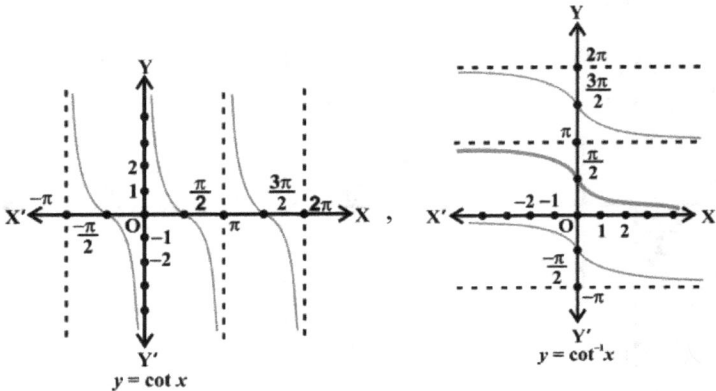

$y = \cot^{-1} x$

Angle of Elevation and Depression

The *angle of elevation* of an object as seen by an observer is the angle between the horizontal and the line from the object to the observer's eye (line of sight). In this case the object is above the level of the observer.

If the object is below the observer, then the angle between the horizontal and the line of sight of the observer is known as the *angle of depression*.

Using trigonometric ratios we can determine the height or length of an object or the distance between two distant objects.

5

Calculus Formulae

LIMIT AND CONTINUITY

In Calculus, a limit is the value that a sequence or function approaches as the input approaches some value.

$\lim\limits_{x\to\bar{a}} f(x)$ is the expected value of f at $x = a$ given the values of f near x to the left of a. This value is called the left hand limit of f at a.

$\lim\limits_{x\to a^+} f(x)$ is the expected value of f at $x = a$ given the values of f near x to the right of a. This value is called the right hand limit of f at a.

If the left hand limit and the right hand limit coincide, we say that value is the limit of the function at that point. If as   , then   is called limit of the function   which is written as

$$\lim\limits_{x\to a} \ (\ ) =$$

Let f and g be two functions such that both $\lim\limits_{x\to a} f(x)$ and $\lim\limits_{x\to a} g(x)$ exist, then

(i) Limit of the sum of two functions is sum of the limits of the functions. $\lim\limits_{x\to a}[f(x)+g(x)] = \lim\limits_{x\to a} f(x) + \lim\limits_{x\to a} g(x)$

(ii) Limit of the difference of two functions is difference of the limits of the functions. $\lim\limits_{x\to a}[f(x)-g(x)] = \lim\limits_{x\to a} f(x) - \lim\limits_{x\to a} g(x)$

(iii) Limit of the product of two functions is product of the limits of the functions. $\lim\limits_{x\to a}[f(x)\cdot g(x)] = \lim\limits_{x\to a} f(x)\cdot \lim\limits_{x\to a} g(x)$

(iv) If g is a constant function such that $= k$ for some real number   then $\lim\limits_{x\to a}[(kf)(x)]$ $k \lim\limits_{x\to a} f(x)$

(v) Limit of the quotient of two functions is quotient of the limits of the functions. $\lim\limits_{x\to a}\dfrac{f(x)}{g(x)} = \dfrac{\lim\limits_{x\to a} f(x)}{\lim\limits_{x\to a} g(x)}$

Limit of a Rational Function

For a rational function $f(x) = \dfrac{g(x)}{h(x)}$ where $g(x)$ and $h(x)$ are ploynomials and $h(x) \neq 0$

$$\lim_{x \to a} f(x) = \lim_{x \to a} \frac{g(x)}{h(x)} = \frac{\lim\limits_{x \to a} g(x)}{\lim\limits_{x \to a} h(x)} = \frac{g(a)}{h(a)}$$

A Standard Limit

For any positive integer n,

$$\lim_{x \to a} \frac{x^n - a^n}{x - a} = na^{n-1}$$

Limits of Trigonometric Functions

(i) Let f and g be two real valued functions with the same domain such that $f(x) \leq g(x)$ for all x in the domain of definition. For some a, if both

$\lim\limits_{x \to a} f(x)$ and $\lim\limits_{x \to a} g(x)$ exist, then $\lim\limits_{x \to a} f(x) \leq \lim\limits_{x \to a} g(x)$.

(ii) *Sandwich Theorem*

Let f, g and h be real functions such that $f(x) \leq g(x) \leq h(x)$ for all x in the common domain of definition. For some real number number a, if $\lim\limits_{x \to a} f(x) = l = \lim\limits_{x \to a} h(x)$, then $\lim\limits_{x \to a} g(x) = l$.

(iii) $\lim\limits_{x \to 0} \dfrac{\sin x}{x} = 1$ (iv) $\lim\limits_{x \to 0} \cos x = 1$

(v) $\lim\limits_{x \to 0} \dfrac{1 - \cos x}{x} = 0$ (vi) $\lim\limits_{x \to 0} \dfrac{\tan x}{x} = 1$

Continuous Function

A function f is continuous at $x = c$ if the function is defined at $x = c$ and if the value of the function at $x = c$ equals the limit of the function at $x = c$.

$$\lim_{x \to c} f(x) = f(c)$$

• A function is continuous if it is continuous on the whole of its domain.

• If f is not continuous at c, we say f is discontinuous at c and c is called a point of discontinuity of f.

Algebra of Continuous Function

If f and g are continuous functions at a real number c, then

(i) $f + g$ is continuous at $x = c$

(ii) $f - g$ is continuous at $x = c$

(iii) $f \cdot g$ is continuous at $x = c$

(iv) $\left(\dfrac{f}{g}\right)$ is continuous at $x = c$ if $g(c) \neq 0$

Let f and g be real valued functions such that $(f \circ g$ c.
If g is continuous at c and if f is continuous at   , then   is
continuous at c.

DIFFERENTIABILITY

A function f is differentiable at a point c in its domain if both

$$\lim_{h \to ^-} \frac{f(c+h)-f(c)}{h} \quad \text{and} \quad \lim_{h \to ^+} \frac{f(c+h)-f(c)}{h}$$

tive of   at c is denoted by

differentiable at every point of [a, b].

f at any point x is given by

$$f'(x) = \frac{d}{dx}(f(x)) = \lim_{h \to} \frac{f(x+h)-f(x)}{h}$$

tives of the functions.

$$\frac{d}{dx}[f(x)+g(x)] = \frac{d}{dx}f(x) + \frac{d}{dx}g(x)$$

the derivatives of the functions.

$$\frac{d}{dx}[f(x)-g(x)] = \frac{d}{dx}f(x) - \frac{d}{dx}g(x)$$

(iii) Product Rule(or Leibnitz Rule)

$$\frac{d}{dx}[f(x) \cdot g(x)] = \frac{d}{dx}f(x) \cdot g(x) + f(x) \cdot \frac{d}{dx}g(x)$$

OR

If $u = f(x)$ and $v = g(x)$, then $(uv)' = u'v + uv'$

(iv) Quotient Rule

$$\frac{d}{dx}\left(\frac{f(x)}{g(x)} \right) = \frac{\frac{d}{dx}f(x) \cdot g(x) - f(x)\frac{d}{dx}g(x)}{(g(x))^2}$$

OR

$$\left(\frac{u}{v} \right)' = \frac{u'v - uv'}{v^2}, \text{ where } u = f(x) \text{ and } v = g(x)$$

Note:

- If a function f is differentiable at a point c, then it is also continuous at that point.
- Every differentiable function is continuous but every continuous function is not differentiable.

Derivative of a Polynomial

Let $f(x) = a_n x^n + a_{n-1} x^{n-1} + \ldots + a_1 x + a^0$ be a polynomial function, where $a_i s$ are all real numbers and $a_n \neq 0$. Then, the derivative function is given by $\dfrac{df(x)}{dx} = n a_n x^{n-1} + (n-1) a_{n-1} x^{x-2} + \ldots + 2 a_2 x + a_1$

Derivative of Some Standard Functions

Function	Derivative
x^n	nx^{n-1}
$\dfrac{1}{x^n}$	$-nx^{-n-1}$
$\sqrt{x}$	$\dfrac{1}{2\sqrt{x}}$
Constant function	0
$sinx$	$cosx$
$cosx$	$-sinx$
$tanx$	sec^2x
e^x	e^x
a^x	$a^x \log_e a$
$\log_e x$	$\dfrac{1}{x}$
$\log_a x$	$\dfrac{1}{x \log_e a}$

Derivatives of Inverse Trigonometric Functions

Function	Derivative	Domain
$sin^{-1}x$	$\dfrac{1}{\sqrt{1-x^2}}$	$x \in (-1,1)$
$cos^{-1}x$	$\dfrac{-1}{\sqrt{1-x^2}}$	$x \in (-1,1)$
$tan^{-1}x$	$\dfrac{1}{1+x^2}$	R
$cot^{-1}x$	$\dfrac{-1}{1+x^2}$	R
$sec^{-1}x$	$\dfrac{1}{x\sqrt{x^2-1}}$	$(-\infty, -1) \cup (1, \infty)$
$cosec^{-1}x$	$\dfrac{-1}{x\sqrt{x^2-1}}$	$(-\infty, -1) \cup (1, \infty)$

Derivative of a Function with Respect to Another Function

If $y = f(x)$ and $z = g(x)$, then the derivative of $f(x)$ with respect to $g(x)$ is

$$\frac{dy}{dz} = \frac{f'(x)}{g'(x)}$$

Logarithmic Differentiation

Logarithmic Differentiation is the process of differentiation of an equation by taking logarithm of both sides.

Case I

$$y = f(x) = [u(x)]^{v(x)}$$

To find the derivative, we find logarithm (to base e) of both sides

$$\log(y) = v(x)\log[u(x)]$$

Next, we differentiate by using the chain rule.

$$\frac{dy}{dx} = y\left[\frac{v(x)}{u(x)} \cdot u'(x) + v'(x) \cdot \log[u(x)]\right]$$

Case II

$$y = \frac{f_1(x)f_2(x)}{g_1(x)g_2(x)}$$

To find the derivative, we find logarithm of both sides and then differentiate with respect to x.

$$\frac{1}{y}\frac{dy}{dx} = \frac{f_1'(x)}{f_1(x)} + \frac{f_2'(x)}{f_2(x)} - \frac{g_1'(x)}{g_1(x)} - \frac{g_2'(x)}{g_2(x)}$$

If $y = \begin{vmatrix} f(x) & g(x) & h(x) \\ p(x) & q(x) & r(x) \\ u(x) & v(x) & w(x) \end{vmatrix}$, then

$$\frac{dy}{dx} = \begin{vmatrix} f'(x) & g'(x) & h'(x) \\ p(x) & q(x) & r(x) \\ u(x) & v(x) & w(x) \end{vmatrix} + \begin{vmatrix} f(x) & g(x) & h(x) \\ p'(x) & q'(x) & r'(x) \\ u(x) & v(x) & w(x) \end{vmatrix} + \begin{vmatrix} f(x) & g(x) & h(x) \\ p(x) & q(x) & r(x) \\ u'(x) & v'(x) & w'(x) \end{vmatrix}$$

If   then

$$y_1 = \frac{dy}{dx} = f'(x)$$

$$y_2 = \frac{d}{dx}\left(\frac{dy}{dx}\right) = \frac{d^2 y}{dx^2} = f''(x)$$

$$y_3 = \frac{d}{dx}\left(\frac{d^2 y}{dx^2}\right) = f'''(x)$$

called successive differentiation.

APPLICATION OF DERIVATIVES

If a physical quantity y varies with another quantity x, satisfying some rule   then

Rate of change of y with respect to $x = f'(x) = \dfrac{dy}{dx}$

Rate of change of y with respect to x at $x = f'(x)$ $\left.\dfrac{dy}{dx}\right]_{x \ x}$

(i) $\dfrac{dy}{dx}$ is positive if y increases as x increases.

(ii) $\dfrac{dy}{dx}$ is negative if y decreases as x increases.

Chain Rule

If two variables x and y vary with respect to another variable t or if   and   then the Chain Rule is given by

$$\frac{dy}{dx} = \frac{dy}{dt} \Big/ \frac{dx}{dt} \qquad \frac{dx}{dt} \neq$$

Let $f : [\quad]$ R be a continuous function on $[\quad]$ and differentiable on $(\quad)$ such that   where a and   are some real numbers then there exists some c in $(\quad)$ such that

Geometric Interpretation of Rolle's Theorem

The slope of the tangent of the curve at various points between a and b is parallel to the x axis.

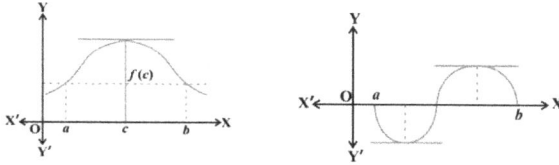

Lagrange's Mean Value Theorem

Let $f : [a,b] \to R$ be a continuous function on $[a,b]$ and differentiable on (a,b), then there exists some c in (a,b) such that

$$f'(c) = \frac{f(b) - f(a)}{b - a}$$

Geometric Interpretation of Mean Value Theorem

The slope of the tangent of the curve at a point $(c, f(c))$ between a and b is parallel to the secant between $(a, f(a))$ and $(b, f(b))$.

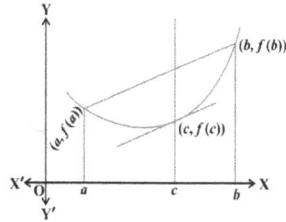

Increasing Function on an Interval

Let I be an open interval contained in the domain of a real valued function f. Then f is said to be

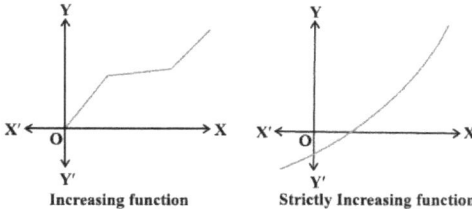

Increasing function   Strictly Increasing function

(i) increasing on I if $x_1 < x_2$ in I $\Rightarrow f(x_1) \leq f(x_2)$ for all $x_1, x_2 \in$ I.
(ii) strictly increasing on I if $x_1 < x_2$ in I $\Rightarrow f(x_1) < f(x_2)$ for all $x_1, x_2 \in$ I.

Decreasing Function on an Interval

Let I be an open interval contained in the domain of a real valued function f. Then f is said to be

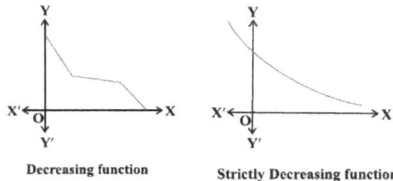

Decreasing function   Strictly Decreasing function

(i) decreasing on I if $x_1 < x_2$ in I $\Rightarrow f(x_1) \geq f(x_2)$ for all $x_1, x_2 \in I$.

(ii) strictly decreasing on I if $x_1 < x_2$ in I $\Rightarrow f(x_1) > f(x_2)$ for all $x_1, x_2 \in I$.

Increasing or Decreasing Function at a Point

Let x_0 be a point in the domain of definition of a real valued function f. Then f is said to be increasing, strictly increasing, decreasing or strictly decreasing at x_0 if there exists an open interval I containing x_0 such that f is increasing, strictly increasing, decreasing or strictly decreasing, respectively, in I.

An Important Theorem

Let the function f be continuous on $[a, b]$ and differentiable on (a,b) then

(a) f is increasing in $[a,b]$ if $f'(x) > 0$ for each $x \in (a, b)$

(b) f is strictly increasing in (a,b) if $f'(x) > 0$ for each $x \in (a, b)$

(c) f is decreasing in $[a,b]$ if $f'(x) < 0$ for each $x \in (a, b)$

(d) f is strictly decreasing in (a,b) if $f'(x) < 0$ for each $x \in (a, b)$

(e) f is a constant function in $[a,b]$ if $f'(x) = 0$ for each $x \in (a, b)$

(f) A function will be increasing (decreasing) in R if it is increasing(decreasing) in every interval of R.

Monotonic Function

If a function f in an interval I is either increasing or decreasing, then it is called a monotonic function.

Equation of Tangent and Normal

Slope of Tangent

(i) For a curve $y = f(x)$ the slope of the tangent at (x_0, y_0) is given by

$$\left[\frac{dy}{dx}\right]_{(x_0, y_0)} \left(\text{or } f'(x_0)\right)$$

(ii) If a tangent line to the curve $y = f(x)$ makes an angle θ in the positive direction, then

Slope of the tangent $= \dfrac{dy}{dx} = \tan\theta$

Note:

If $\theta = 0°$, the tangent is parallel to the x-axis.

If $\theta \to 90°$, the tangent is perpendicular to the x-axis (parallel to the y axis).

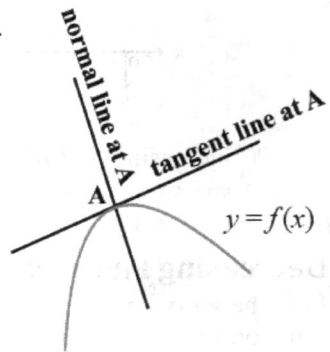

Mathematics Formulae

Equation of Tangent

Equation of the tangent to the curve $y = f(x)$ at (x_0, y_0) is

$$y - y_0 = f'(x_0)(x - x_0)$$

Note:

- If $\theta = 0°$, the equation of the tangent at (x_0, y_0) is given by $y = y_0$.
- If $\theta \rightarrow 90°$, the equation of the tangent at (x_0, y_0) is given by $x = x_0$.
- Two curves intersect at right angle if the tangents to the curves at the point of intersection are perpendicular to each other.

Slope of Normal

For a curve $y = f(x)$, the slope of the normal at (x_0, y_0) is given by

$$\frac{-1}{f'(x_0)} \text{ if } f'(x_0) \neq 0$$

Equation of Normal

Equation of the normal to the curve $y = f(x)$ at (x_0, y_0) is

$$y - y_0 = \frac{-1}{f'(x_0)}(x - x_0)$$

Note:

- If $\theta = 0°$, the equation of the normal at (x_0, y_0) is given by $x = x_0$.
- If $\theta \rightarrow 90°$, the equation of the normal at (x_0, y_0) is given by $y = y_0$.

Approximation

The differential of the independent variable is equal to the increment of the variable and the differential of the dependent variable is not equal to the increment of the variable.

Let $y = f(x)$, Δx denote a small increment in x and Δy a small increment in y. The increment in y corresponding to the increment in x is given by $\Delta y = f(x + \Delta x) - f(x)$.

(i)   The differential of x represented by dx, is given by $dx = \Delta x$
(ii) The differential of y represented by dy is given by

$$dy = f'(x)dx \text{ or } dy = \left(\frac{dy}{dx}\right)\Delta x$$

Maximum, Minimum or Extreme Value

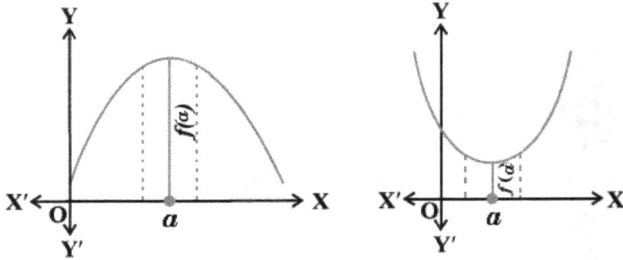

Let f be a function defined on an interval I, then

(i) f is said to have a maximum value in I, if there exists a point a in I such that $f(a) \geq f(x)$, for all $x \in$ I.

$f(a)$ is called the maximum value of f in I and the point a is called a *point of maximum* value of f in I.

(ii) f is said to have a minimum value in I, if there exists a point a in I such that $f(a) \leq f(x)$, for all $x \in$ I.

$f(a)$ is called the minimum value of f in I and the point a, is called a *point of minimum* value of f in I.

(iii) f is said to have an extreme value in I if there exists a point a in I such that $f(a)$ is either a maximum value or a minimum value of f in I.

In this case, $f(a)$ is called an extreme value of f in I and the point a is called an *extreme point.*

Note:

- Every monotonic function assumes its maximum/minimum value at the end points of the domain of definition of the function.
- Every continuous function on a closed interval has a maximum and a minimum value.

Turning Point

The point where the graph of a function changes its nature from increasing to decreasing or vice versa is known as the turning point (or point of inflection) of the function.

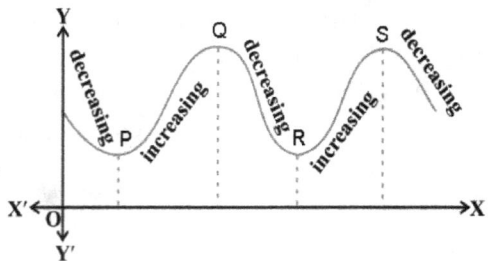

Local Maxima and Local Minima

Let f be a real valued function and let a be an interior point in the domain of f, then

(i) a is called a point of local maxima if there is an $h > 0$ such that
$f(a) \geq f(x)$, for all $x \in (a - h, a + h)$.
The value $f(c)$ is called the *local maximum* value of f.

(ii) a is called a point of local minima if there is an $h > 0$ such that
$f(a) \leq f(x)$, for all x in $(a - h, a + h)$
The value $f(a)$ is called the *local minimum* value of f.

Geometric Interpretation

- If $x = a$ is a point of local maxima of f, the function f is increasing in the interval $(a - h, a)$ and decreasing in the interval $(a, a + h)$. Hence $f'(a) = 0$.
- If $x = a$ is a point of local minima of f, the function f is decreasing in the interval $(a - h, a)$ and increasing in the interval $(a, a + h)$. Hence $f'(a) = 0$.

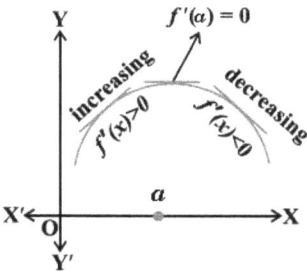

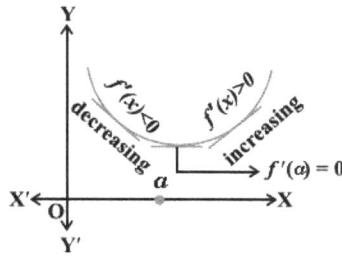

An Important Theorem

Let f be a function defined on an open interval I and let $a \in$ I be any point. If f has a local maxima or a local minima at $x = a$, then either $f'(a) = 0$ or f is not differentiable at a.

Critical Point

A point a in the domain of a function f at which either $f'(a) = 0$ or f is not differentiable is called a critical point of f.

If f is continuous at a and $f'(a) = 0$, then there exists an $h > 0$ such that f is differentiable in the interval $(a - h, a + h)$.

Absolute Maxima and Absolute Minima

(i) Let f be a continuous function on a closed interval I, then f has the absolute maximum and absolute minimum value and f attains them at least once in I.

(ii) Let f be a differentiable function on a closed interval I and let a be any interior point of I. Then
   (a) $f'(a) = 0$ if, f attains its absolute maximum value at a.
   (b) $f'(a) = 0$ if, f attains its absolute minimum value at a.

Method to Find Absolute Maxima or Minima

(i) For the function $y = f(x)$, find $f'(x)$.
(ii) Find points x where either $f'(x) = 0$ or f is not differentiable. These points are called the critical points of f in the interval.
(iii)Take the end points of the interval.
(iv)At the end points and the critical points, calculate the values of f.
(v) Identify the maximum and minimum values of f in the above step. This maximum value will be the absolute maximum value of f and the minimum value will be the absolute minimum value of f.

First Derivative Test

Let f be a function defined on an open interval I. Let f be continuous at a critical point a in I, then

(i) If $f'(x)$ changes sign from positive to negative as x increases through a, i.e., if $f'(x) > 0$ at every point sufficiently close to and to the left of a, and $f'(x) < 0$ at every point sufficiently close to and to the right of a, then a is a point of local maxima.

(ii) If $f'(x)$ changes sign from negative to positive as x increases through a, i.e., if $f'(x) < 0$ at every point sufficiently close to and to the left of a, and $f'(x) > 0$ at every point sufficiently close to and to the right of a, then a is a point of local minima.

(iii)If $f'(x)$ does not change sign as x increases through a, then a is neither a point of local maxima nor a point of local minima. Such a point is called point of inflection.

Second Derivative Test

Let f be a function defined on an interval I and $a \in I$. Let f be twice differentiable at a, then

(i) $x = a$ is a point of local maxima if $f'(a) = 0$ and $f''(a) < 0$
   The value $f(a)$ is local maximum value of f.
(ii) $x = a$ is a point of local minima if $f'(a) = 0$ and $f''(a) > 0$
   The value of $f(a)$ is local minimum value of f.
(iii)The test fails if $f'(a) = 0$ and $f''(a) = 0$.

Mathematics Formulae

INDEFINITE INTEGRAL

The inverse process of differentiation is called integration. The proc-

called integration.

If there is a function F such that

$$\frac{d}{dx}F(x) = f(x), \quad x \quad \text{I (interval), then}$$

$$\frac{d}{dx}[F(x) + C] = f(x), x \in 1$$

where C is any arbitrary real number.

f with respect to x is repre-

sented by $\int f(x)dx = F(x) + C$

where C is any arbitrary real number known as the constant of integration.

Symbols and Meanings

Symbols/Terms	Meaning
$\int f(x)dx$	Integral of f with respect to x
x in $\int f(x)dx$	Variable of integration
$f(x)$ in $\int f(x)dx$	Integrand
An integral of f	A function F such that F'(x) =

Geometric Interpretation of Indefinite Integral

lection of family of curves each of which is obtained by translating one of the curves parallel to itself upwards or downwards along the y axis.

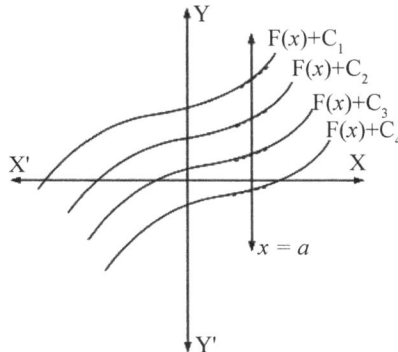

Properties of Indefinite Integral

(i) The process of differentiation and integration are inverse of each other.

$$\frac{d}{dx}\int f(x)dx = f(x) \text{ and } \int f'(x)dx = f(x) + C,$$

where C is any arbitrary constant.

(ii) Two indefinite integrals with the same derivative lead to the same family of curves and so they are equivalent.

If f and g are two functions such that $\frac{d}{dx}\int f(x)dx = \frac{d}{dx}\int g(x)dx$

then $\int f(x)dx$ and $\int g(x)dx$ are equivalent.

(iii) For any real number k, $\int k f(x)dx = k\int f(x)dx$

(iv) $\int [f(x) + g(x)]dx = \int f(x)dx + \int g(x)dx$

(v) $\int [k_1 f_1(x) + k_2 f_2(x) + ... + k_n f_n(x)]dx$

$= k_1\int f_1(x)dx + k_2\int f_2(x)dx + ... + k_n\int f_n(x)dx$

where $f_1, f_2, ..., f_n$ are finite functions of x and $k_1, k_2, ... k_n$ are real numbers.

Some Standard Integrals

No.	Derivatives	Integrals (Anti derivatives)
(i)	$\frac{d}{dx}\left(\frac{x^{n+1}}{n+1}\right) = x^n$ Particularly, we note that $\frac{d}{dx}(x) = 1$	$\int x^n dx = \frac{x^{n+1}}{n+1} + C, n \neq -1$ $\int dx = x + C$
(ii)	$\frac{d}{dx}(\sin x) = \cos x$	$\int \cos x\, dx = \sin x + C$
(iii)	$\frac{d}{dx}(-\cos x) = \sin x$	$\int \sin x\, dx = -\cos x + C$
(iv)	$\frac{d}{dx}(\tan x) = \sec^2 x$	$\int \sec^2 x\, dx = \tan x + C$
(v)	$\frac{d}{dx}(-\cot x) = \operatorname{cosec}^2 x$	$\int \operatorname{cosec}^2 x\, dx = -\cot x = C$
(vi)	$\frac{d}{dx}(\sec x) = \sec x \tan x$	$\int \sec x \tan x\, dx = \sec x + C$
(vii)	$\frac{d}{dx}(-\operatorname{cosec} x) = \operatorname{cosec} x \cot x$	$\int \operatorname{cosec} x \cot x\, dx = -\operatorname{cosec} x + C$

Mathematics Formulae

(viii)	$\dfrac{d}{dx}(\sin^{-1}x) = \dfrac{1}{\sqrt{1-x^2}}$	$\displaystyle\int \dfrac{dx}{\sqrt{1-x^2}} = \sin^{-1}x + C$
(ix)	$\dfrac{d}{dx}(-\cos^{-1}x) = \dfrac{1}{\sqrt{1-x^2}}$;	$\displaystyle\int \dfrac{dx}{\sqrt{1-x^2}} = -\cos^{-1}x + C$
(x)	$\dfrac{d}{dx}(\tan^{-1}x) = \dfrac{1}{1+x^2}$;	$\displaystyle\int \dfrac{dx}{1+x^2} = \tan^{-1}x + C$
(xi)	$\dfrac{d}{dx}(-\cot^{-1}x) = \dfrac{1}{1+x^2}$	$\displaystyle\int \dfrac{dx}{1+x^2} = -\cot^{-1}x + C$
(xii)	$\dfrac{d}{dx}(\sec^{-1}x) = \dfrac{1}{x\sqrt{x^2-1}}$;	$\displaystyle\int \dfrac{dx}{x\sqrt{x^2-1}} = \sec^{-1}x + C$
(xiii)	$\dfrac{d}{dx}(-\mathrm{cosec}^{-1}x) = \dfrac{1}{x\sqrt{x^2-1}}$;	$\displaystyle\int \dfrac{dx}{x\sqrt{x^2-1}} = -\mathrm{cosec}^{-1}x + C$
(xiv)	$\dfrac{d}{dx}(e^x) = e^x$	$\displaystyle\int e^x\,dx = e^x + C$
(xv)	$\dfrac{d}{dx}(\log|x|) = \dfrac{1}{x}$	$\displaystyle\int \dfrac{1}{x}\,dx = \log|x| + C$
(xvi)	$\dfrac{d}{dx}\left(\dfrac{a^x}{\log a}\right) = a^x$	$\displaystyle\int a^x\,dx = \dfrac{a^x}{\log a} + C$

Integrals of Some Particular Functions

(i) $\displaystyle\int \dfrac{dx}{x^2-a^2} = \dfrac{1}{2a}\log\left|\dfrac{x-a}{x+a}\right| + C$

(ii) $\displaystyle\int \dfrac{dx}{a^2-x^2} = \dfrac{1}{2a}\log\left|\dfrac{a+x}{a-x}\right| + C$

(iii) $\displaystyle\int \dfrac{dx}{x^2+a^2} = \dfrac{1}{a}\tan^{-1}\dfrac{x}{a} + C$

(iv) $\displaystyle\int \dfrac{dx}{\sqrt{x^2-a^2}} = \log\left|x + \sqrt{x^2-a^2}\right| + C$

(v) $\displaystyle\int \dfrac{dx}{\sqrt{a^2-x^2}} = \sin^{-1}\dfrac{x}{a} + C$

(vi) $\displaystyle\int \dfrac{dx}{\sqrt{x^2+a^2}} = \log\left|x + \sqrt{x^2+a^2}\right| + C$

(vii) To find the integral $\displaystyle\int \dfrac{dx}{ax^2+bx+c}$, complete the square of the quadratic expression $ax^2 + bx + c$

$$ax^2 + bx + c = a\left[x^2 + \dfrac{b}{a}x + \dfrac{c}{a}\right] = a\left[\left(x + \dfrac{b}{2a}\right)^2 + \left(\dfrac{c}{a} - \dfrac{b^2}{4a^2}\right)\right]$$

Substitute $x + \dfrac{b}{2a} = t$ so that $dx = dt$, Put $\dfrac{c}{a} - \dfrac{b^2}{4a^2} = \pm k^2$

Depending upon the sign of $\left(\dfrac{c}{a} - \dfrac{b^2}{4a^2}\right)$ the integral is reduced to

$\dfrac{1}{a}\int\dfrac{dt}{t^2 \pm k^2}$ which can easily be solved.

(viii) To find the integral of the type $\int\dfrac{dx}{\sqrt{ax^2 + bx + c}}$, use 4, 6 and 7 as mentioned above.

(ix) To find the integral of the type $\int\dfrac{px + q}{ax^2 + bx + c}dx$, where p, q, a, b, c are constants. We find real numbers A, B such that

$$px + q = A\dfrac{d}{dx}(ax^2 + bx + c) + B = A(2ax + b)B$$

We can find the values of A and B by equating the coefficients of x and the constant terms and solving the equation. By substituting the value of A and B, the given integral reduces to some known form.

(x) For the evaluation of the integral of the type $\int\dfrac{(px + q)dx}{\sqrt{ax^2 + bx + c}}$ proceed as in 9 and transform the integral into one of the known forms.

Methods of Integration

Substitution Method

By changing the independent variable x to t using the substitution $x = g(t)$ the integral $\int f(x)dx$ can be transformed into another form which is some standard integral or sum of standard integrals.

$$I = \int f(x)dx$$

Substitute $x = g(t)$

$$\dfrac{dx}{dt} = g'(t)$$

$$I = \int f(x)dx = \int f(g(t))g'(t)dt$$

Special Integrals Obtained by Substitution Method

(i) $\int \tan x\, dx = \log|\sec x| + C$

(ii) $\int \cot x\, dx = \log|\sin x| + C$

(iii) $\int \sec x\, dx = \log|\sec x + \tan x| + C$

(iv) $\int \operatorname{cosec} x\, dx = \log|\operatorname{cosec} x - \cot x| + C$

Partial Fraction Method

If $P(x)$ and $Q(x)$ are two polynomials such that $Q(x) \neq 0$, then to solve the following integral we have two cases:

$$\int \frac{P(x)}{Q(x)} dx$$

Case I

a) If $\dfrac{P(x)}{Q(x)}$ is an improper rational function, divide $P(x)$ by $Q(x)$.

$\dfrac{P(x)}{Q(x)} = T(x) + \dfrac{R(x)}{Q(x)}$ where $T(x)$ is the quotient and $R(x)$ is the remainder

b) Write $\dfrac{R(x)}{Q(x)}$ as partial fraction expansion.

c) Integrate $T(x)$ and the partial fraction expansion.

Case II

a) If $\dfrac{P(x)}{Q(x)}$ is a proper rational function, write it as partial fracion expansion.

b) Integrate the partial fraction expansion.

Integration by Parts

If *f(x)* is the first function and *g(x)* is the second function, then

$$\int f(x)g(x)dx = f(x)\int g(x)dx - \int [f'(x)\int g(x)dx]dx$$

The integral of the product of two functions
= (first function) × (integral of the second function) − Integral of [(differential coefficient of the first function) × (integral of the second function)]

- Product of any two given functions cannot be solved by integration by parts. (This method is applicable only for some functions).
- Generally inverse trigonometric function, logarithmic function and polynomial function are taken as the first function.

Special integrals obtained by integration by parts

1. $\int \sqrt{x^2 - a^2}\, dx = \dfrac{x}{2}\sqrt{x^2 - a^2} - \dfrac{a^2}{2} \log\left|x + \sqrt{x^2 - a^2}\right| + C$

2. $\int \sqrt{x^2 + a^2}\, dx = \dfrac{1}{2}x\sqrt{x^2 + a^2} + \dfrac{a^2}{2} \log\left|x + \sqrt{x^2 + a^2}\right| + C$

3. $\int \sqrt{a^2 - x^2}\, dx = \dfrac{1}{2}x\sqrt{a^2 - x^2} + \dfrac{a^2}{2} \sin^{-1}\dfrac{x}{a} + C$

4. $\int e^x[f(x) + f'(x)]dx = e^x f(x) + C$

DEFINITE INTEGRAL

Let f] and
F be an anti derivative of f. Then

$$\int_a () = [F( )]_a = F( ) - F( )$$

f over [ ] where a is the lower limit of the integral and is the upper limit of the integral.

Note:

Definite Integral as Limit of Sum

$$\int_a () = (-) \lim_{n \to \infty} \frac{1}{n} [( )+ (+)+ + (+(-1))]$$

where $h = \dfrac{-}{n} \to$ as $n \to \infty$

Difference Method

$$\int f(x)dx .$$ Let this be $F(x)$.

(iii)Calculate F(b) – F(a).

(iv) $\int_a () = F( ) - F( )$

Substitution Method

(i) Consider the integral without limits and substitute, $f(x) = t$ to reduce the given integral to a known form.

(ii) Integrate the new integrand with respect to the new variable (Ignore the constant of integration).

(iii)Substitute back for the new variable and write the answer in terms of the original variable.

(iv)Find the values of answers obtained in (iii) at the given limits

lower limit.

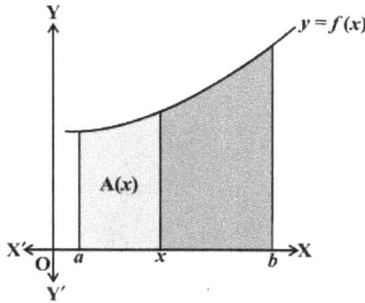

Area Function

Area function A(x) is given by

$$A(x) = \int_a^x f(x)dx$$

where $f(x) > 0$ for all $x \in [a, b]$.

First Fundamental Theorem of Integral Calculus

Let f be a continuous function on the closed interval $[a, b]$ and let $A(x)$ be the area function. Then
$A'(x) = f(x)$ for all $x \in [a, b]$.

Properties of Definite Integral

(i) $\int_a^b f(x)dx = \int_a^b f(t)dt$

(ii) $\int_a^b f(x)dx = -\int_b^a f(x)dx$

(iii) $\int_a^a f(x)dx = 0$

(iv) $\int_a^b f(x)dx = \int_a^c f(x)dx + \int_c^b f(x)dx$

(v) $\int_a^b f(x)dx = \int_a^b f(a+b-x)dx$

(vi) $\int_0^a f(x)dx = \int_0^a f(a-x)dx$

(vii) $\int_0^{2a} f(x)dx = \int_0^a f(x)dx + \int_0^a f(2a-x)dx$

(viii) $\int_0^{2a} f(x)dx = 2\int_0^a f(x)dx$ if $f(2a-x)=f(x)$ and 0 if $f(2a-x)=-f(x)$

(ix) (a) $\int_{-a}^a f(x)dx = 2\int_0^a f(x)dx$, if f is an even function, i.e., if $f(-x)=f(x)$

(b) $\int_{-a}^a f(x)dx = 0$, if f is an odd function, i.e., if $f(-x) = -f(x)$

APPLICATION OF INTEGRALS

Case I

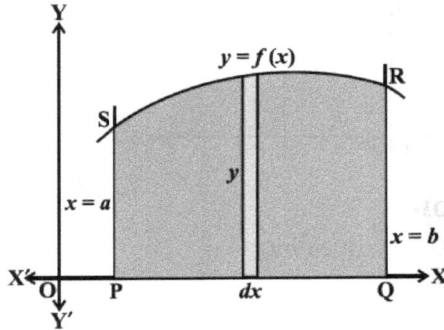

Elementary area

The area of an arbitrary strip of width dx and height y is given by

$dA = ydx$ where $y =$

Total area

The area bounded by the curve x-axis and the ordinates

$x = a$ and   ($> a$) is given by

Total Area = Sum of elementary areas across PQRSP

$$A = \int_a dA = \int_a ydx = \int_a f(x)dx$$

Case II

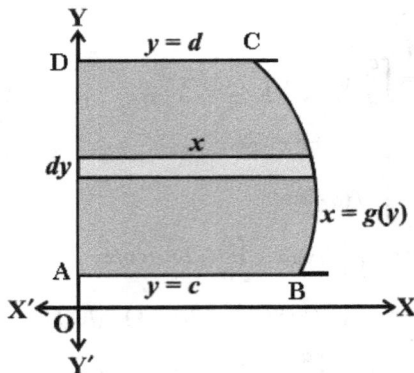

Elementary area

The area of an arbitrary strip of width dy and length x is given by

$dA = xdy$ where $x = g$

Total area

The area bounded by the curve $x = g(y)$, y-axis and the lines $y = c$ and $y = d$ is given by

Total Area = Sum of elementary areas across ABCDA

$$A = \int_c^b x\,dy = \int_c^d g(y)\,dy$$

Area of Curve Below X-Axis

The area bounded by the curve $y = f(x)$ where $f(x) < 0$, x-axis and the ordinates $x = a$ and $x = b$ $(b > a)$ is given by $\left| \int_a^b f(x)\,dx \right|$

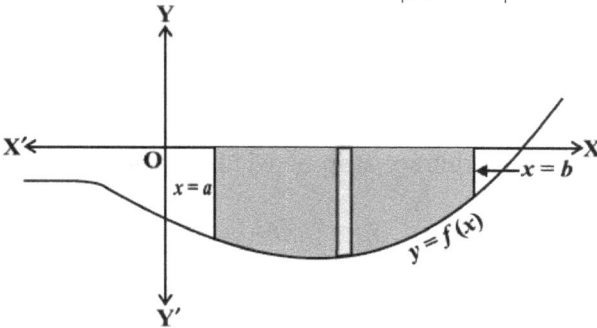

Area of the Curve (Partly Above A-Axis and Partly Below)

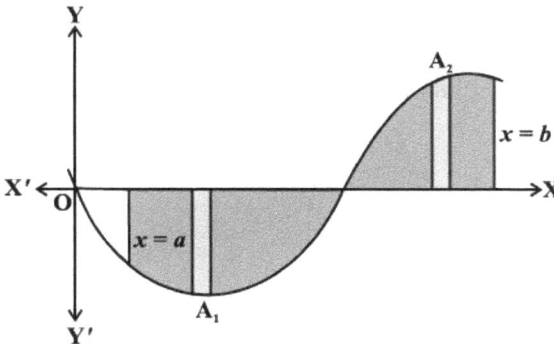

The area $A(A_1 + A_2)$ where $A_1 < 0$, $A_2 > 0$ bounded by the curve $y = f(x)$, x-axis and the ordinates $x = a$ and $x = b$ $(b > a)$ is given by

$$A = |A_1| + A_2$$

Area Bounded by a Curve and a Line

Area bounded by a line and a parabola or a line and a circle or a line and an ellipse is calculated by taking either vertical strips or horizontal strips and integrating them using suitable limits of integration.

Area Between Curves

Case I

Elementary area

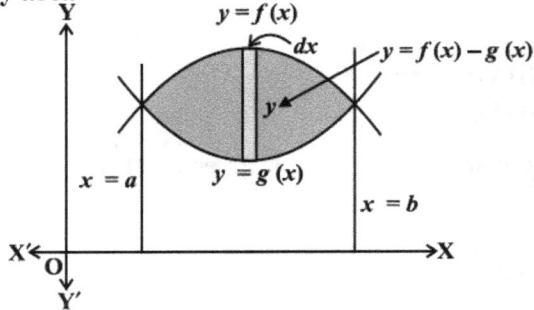

The area of an arbitrary strip of width dx and height $f(x) - g(x)$ is given by

$$dA = [f(x) - g(x)]dx$$

Total area

The area of the region enclosed between two curves $y = f(x)$, $y = g(x)$ where $f(x) \geq g(x)$ in $[a,b]$ and the ordinates $x = a$ and $x = b$ $(b > a)$ is given by

$$A = \int_a^b [f(x) - g(x)]dx$$

Case II

If $f(x) \geq g(x)$ in $[a,c]$ and $f(x) \leq g(x)$ in $[c, b]$ where $a < c < b$, then

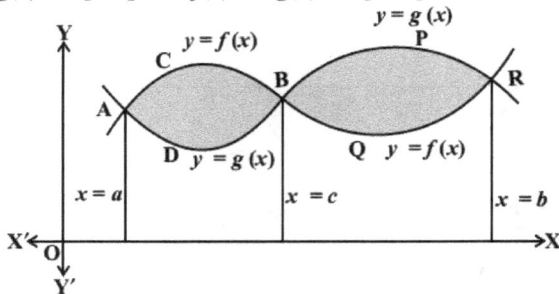

the area of the region bounded by $f(x)$ and $g(x)$ is given by

Total Area = Area of ADBCA + BQRPB

Total Area $= \int_a^c [f(x) - g(x)]dx + \int_c^b [g(x) - f(x)]dx$

DIFFERENTIAL EQUATION

ent variable with respect to the independent variable. For example,

$$x\frac{dy}{dx} + y =$$

In the above differential equation, y is the dependent variable and x is the independent variable.

A differential equation involving derivatives of the dependent variable with respect to only one independent variable is called an ordinary differential equation.

$$\frac{d^2y}{dx^2} + \left(\frac{dy}{dx}\right)^3 =$$

Order of a Differential Equation

Order of a differential equation is the order of the highest order derivative occurring in the differential equation.

independent parameters and not equal to the number of all the parameters in a family of curves.

Degree of a Differential Equation

equation in its derivatives.

power of the highest order derivative in it.

Note:

ways positive integers.

Solution of a Differential Equation

called its solution.

der of the differential equation is called a general solution.

lution.

are the number of arbitrary constants in the given function.

Formation of Differential Equation Representing a Family of Curves

Case I (One Parameter)

(i) Write the family of curves (F_1) depending on only one parameter in the following form

$$F_1(x, y, a) = 0$$

(ii) Differentiate the above equation with respect to x.

$$g(x, y, y', a) = 0$$

(iii) Obtain the differential equation by eliminating a from the above two equations.

$$F(x, y, y') = 0$$

Case II (Two Parameters)

(i) Write the family of curves (F_2) depending on two parameters say a, b in the following form

$$F_2(x, y, a, b) = 0$$

(ii) Differentiate the above equation with respect to x.

$$g(x, y, y', a, b) = 0$$

(iii) Differentiate the equation obtained in step 2 with respect to x.

$$h(x, y, y', y'', a, b) = 0$$

(iv) Obtain the differential equation by eliminating a and b from the above three equations.

$$F(x, y, y', y'') = 0$$

Variable Separable Method

This method is used to solve such a differential equation in which variables can be separated completely (terms containing y remain with dy and terms containing x remain with dx).

For a differential equation $H(y) = G(x) + C$ where C is an arbitrary constant, $G(x)$ is the anti derivative of $g(x)$ and $H(y)$ is the anti derivative of $1/h(y)$ the solution is given by

$$\int \frac{1}{h(y)} dy = \int g(x) dx + C$$

Note: Depending on the problem, the constant of integration can be taken as C, log C or $\tan^{-1} C$.

Homogeneous Function

A function $F(x, y)$ is said to be homogeneous function of degree n if $F(\lambda x, \lambda y) = \lambda^n F(x, y)$ for any non zero constant λ.

Homogeneous Differential Equation

A differential equation which can be expressed in the form

$$\frac{dy}{dx} = F(x, y) \text{ or } \frac{dy}{dx} = F(x, y)$$

is said to be a homogenous differential equation if F (x,y) is a homogenous function of degree zero.

Solution of Homogeneous Differential Equation

(i) Write the given differential equation in the standard form of

$$\frac{dy}{dx} = F(x, y) = g\left(\frac{y}{x}\right)$$

(ii) Put $y = vx$ and differentiate with respect to x.

(iii) Substitute the value of $\frac{dy}{dx}$ in the given differential equation.

We get $x\frac{dv}{dx} = g(v) - v$

(iv) Separate the variables and integrate both sides to get a solution.

$$\int \frac{dv}{g(v) - v} = \int \frac{1}{x} dx + C$$

(v) Replace v by $\frac{y}{x}$

Note:

If the differential equation is of the form $\frac{dy}{dx} = F(x, y)$, put $x = vy$ and proceed as in the above case.

Linear Differential Equation

A differential equation in which the dependent variable and its differential coefficients occur only in the first degree and are not multiplied together is called a linear differential equation.

It is of the form

$$\frac{dy}{dx} + Py = Q$$

where P and Q are constants or functions of x only. It can also be of the form

$$\frac{dy}{dx} + P_1 x = Q_1$$

where P_1 and Q_1 are constants or functions of y only.

Solution of Linear Differential Equation
Case I

(i) Write the given differential equation in the standard form i.e. $\frac{dy}{dx} + Py = Q$ where P and Q are constants or functions of x only.

(ii) Find the integrating factor (I.F) by

$$\text{I.F} = e^{\int P dx}$$

(iii) Find the solution of the given differential equation by solving the following equation:

$$y(\text{I.F}) = \int (Q \times \text{I.F}) dx + C \text{ where } C \text{ is the constant of integration.}$$

Case II

(i) Write the given differential equation in the standard form $\dfrac{dx}{dy} + P_1 x = Q_1$ where P_1 and Q_1 are constants or functions of y only.

(ii) Find the integrating factor (I.F) by

$$\text{I.F} = e^{\int P_1 dy}$$

(iii) Find the solution of the given differential equation by solving the following equation.

$$x \cdot (\text{I.F}) = \int (Q_1 \times \text{I.F}) dy + C$$

where C is the constant of integration.

Non Linear Differential Equation

A differential equation is non linear differential equation if:

(i) Any of the differential coefficients has exponent more than one.

(ii) The degree of the differential equation is more than one.

(iii) Products containing dependent variable and its differential coefficients are present.

(iv) Exponent of the dependent variable is more than one.

6

Coordinate Geometry Formulae

MENSURATION

Name of Shape	Shape	Formula
Square		Perimeter $= 4 \times s$ Area $= s \times s$
Rectangle		Perimeter $2\ell + 2w$ Area $= \ell \times w$
Parallelogram		Perimeter $= 2\ell + 2b$ Area $=$ base $\times$ height
Rhombus		Perimeter $= 4 \times a$ Area $= (d_1 \times d_2)$
Triangle		Perimeter $= a + b + c$ Area $= (b \times$
Triangle		Perimeter $= 3 \times a$ Area $= (\ 3a^2$
Trapezoid		Perimeter $=$ sum of all sides Area $= (a + b)$ x
Circle		Circumference $= 2 \times \ \times r$ Area $=\ \times r^2$
Semicircle		Circumference $=\ \times r \times$ Area $= (\ r^2)/2$

Useful Formula for Fencing Problems

Length of the fence = Total cost of fencing ÷ Rate

Heron's Formula

Area of Triangle

If a, b, c are three sides of a triangle, then area of triangle by Heron's formula is given by

Area of triangle = $\sqrt{s(s-a)(s-b)(s-c)}$ where $s = \dfrac{a+b+c}{2}$

Area of Quadrilateral

Area of a quadrilateral whose one diagonal and the sides are given, can be calculated by dividing the quadrilateral into two triangles and using the Heron's formula.

Area and Length of a Sector

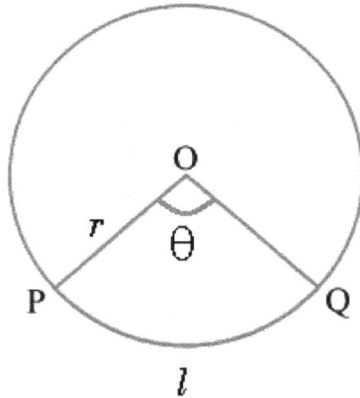

If r is the radius of a circle and θ is the sector angle, then the area of the sectors and the length of the arc are given by

Area of minor sector = $\dfrac{\theta}{360} \times \pi r^2$

Area of major sector = πr^2 – Area of minor sector

Length of arc = $\dfrac{\theta}{360} \times 2\pi r$

Area of a Segment

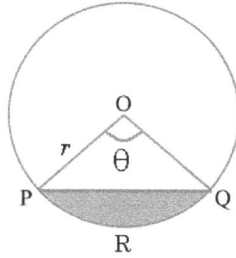

If r is the radius of a circle and θ is the sector angle, then the area of the minor segment is given by

Area of minor segment PRQ

= Area of minor sector OPRQ – Area of triangle POQ

Area of major segment = πr^2 – Area of minor segment

Area and Volume of Cube and Cuboid

S. No.	Name	Figure	Total Surface Area (sq.units)	Curved Surface Area (sq.units)	Volume (cu.units)
1.	Cube		$6a^2$	$4a^2$	a^3 Diagonal $= \sqrt{3}\,a$
2.	Cuboid		$2(lb + bh + hl)$	$2h(l + b)$	$l \times b \times h$ Diagonal $= \sqrt{l^2 + b^2 + h^2}$

Area and Volume of Cylinder, Cone, Sphere and Hemisphere

S. No.	Name	Figure	Lateral or Curved Surface Area (sq. units)	Total Surface Area (sq. units)	Volume (cu. units)
1.	Solid right circular cylinder		$2\pi rh$	$2\pi r(h + r)$	$\pi r^2 h$
2.	Right circular hollow cylinder		$2\pi h(R + r)$	$2\pi h(R + r)$ $(R - r + h)$	$\pi R^2 h - \pi r^2 h$ $\pi h(R^2 - r^2)$ $\pi h(R + r)(R - r)$

3.	Solid right circular cone		$\pi r l$	$\pi r(l + r)$	$\dfrac{1}{3}\pi r^2 h$
4.	Frustum		$\pi l(R + r)$	$\pi l(R + r)$ $+ \pi(R^2 + r^2)$ $l = $ $\sqrt{h^2 + (R - r)^2}$	$\dfrac{1}{3}\pi h(R^2 + r^2 + Rr)$
5.	Sphere		$4\pi r^2$	---	$\dfrac{4}{3}\pi r^3$
6.	Hollow sphere		...	...	$\dfrac{4}{3}\pi(R^3 - r^3)$
7.	Solid Hemishere		$2\pi r^2$	$3\pi r^2$	$\dfrac{2}{3}\pi r^3$
8.	Hollow Hemishere		$2\pi(R^2 + r^2)$	$2\pi(R^2 + r^2)$ $+ \pi(R^2 - r^2)$	$\dfrac{2}{3}\pi(R^3 - r^3)$

9.	A sector of a circle converted into a Cone CSA of cone = Area of sector $$\pi r l = \frac{\theta}{360} \times \pi r^2$$ Length of the sector = Base circumference of the cone $$l = \sqrt{h^2 + r^2}$$ $$h = \sqrt{l^2 - r^2}$$ $$r = \sqrt{l^2 - h^2}$$	10. Volume of water flows out through a pipe = {Cross section area × Speed × Time} 11. No. of new solids obtained by recasting $$= \frac{\text{Volume of the solid which is melted}}{\text{volume of one solid which is made}}$$

12.	Conversions 1m³ = 1000 litres, 1m³ = 1 litre, 1000 cm³ = 1 litre, 1000 litres = 1kl

BASICS OF COORDINATE GEOMETRY

To locate the position of a point in a plane, we require two perpendicular lines. One of them is horizontal and the other is vertical.

The plane is called the **Cartesian plane** or the **coordinate plane** and the lines are known as the axes. The horizontal line is known as the x axis and the vertical line is known as the y axis.

The point where the x axis and y axis intersect is known as the **origin**.

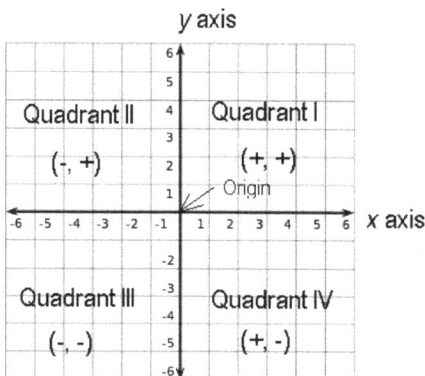

Two numbers written in a certain order are known as an **ordered pair**. For example, while writing the coordinates of any point in cartesian plane(coordinate plane) we write the x
then the y-coordinate i.e. in the form of (   ). x coordinate is known as **abscissa** and the y coordinate is known as **ordinate**.

$$) = (\quad) \text{ if } x = y$$
$$) \text{ if } x \quad y$$

$$x\text{-axis} = (x \qquad x$$
$$y \qquad y \qquad y)$$

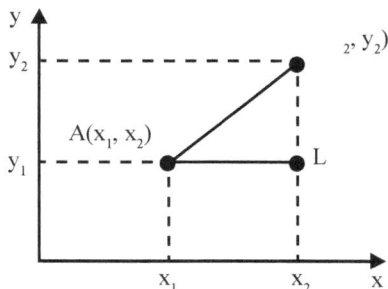

The distance between two points A (x_1, y_1) and B(x_2, y_2) is given by:

$$AB = \sqrt{(x_2 - x_1)^2 + (y_2 - y_1)^2}$$

Distance from Origin

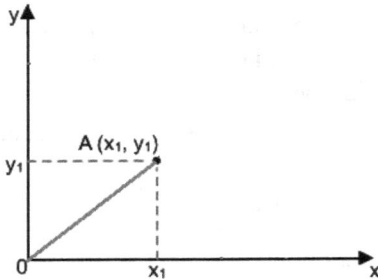

The distance of the point A (x_1, y_1) from the origin is given by:

$$OA = \sqrt{x_1^2 + y_1^2}$$

Mid Point Formula

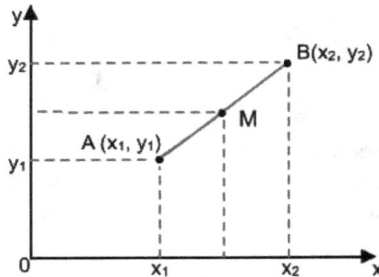

The mid point M of the line segment joining A (x_1, y_1) and B(x_2, y_2) is given by:

$$\left(\frac{x_1 + x_2}{2}, \frac{y_1 + y_2}{2} \right)$$

Section Formula

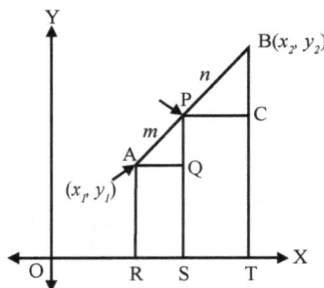

The coordinates of the point P(x,y) which divides the line segment

Mathematics Formulae

joining the points A $(x_1, y_1$ $x_2, y_2)$ in the ratio m: n is given by:

$$\left(\frac{mx_2 + nx_1}{m+n}, \frac{my_2 + my_1}{m+n} \right)$$

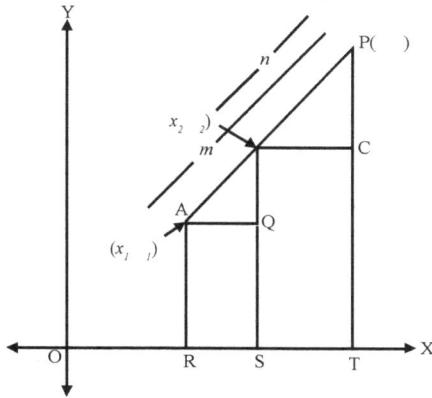

The coordinates of the point P( ) which divides the line segment joining the points A $(x_1, y_1$ $x_2, y_2)$ in the ratio m: n is given by

$$\left(\frac{mx_2 - nx_1}{m-n}, \frac{my_2 - ny_1}{m-n} \right)$$

The area of the triangle formed by the points A $(x_1, y_1$ $x_2, y_2)$ and C (x_3, y_3) is given by the numerical value of the expression:

$$\frac{1}{2}[x_1(y_2 - y_3) + x_2(y_3 - y_1) + x_3(y_1 - y_2)]$$

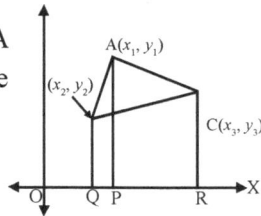

STRAIGHT LINE

forms two angles with the x-axis which are supplementary.

with positive direction of x-axis and measured anti clockwise is called the **inclination of the line**

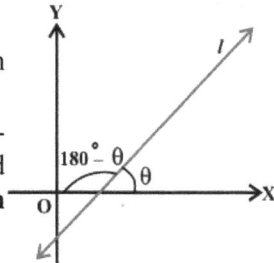

inciding with x axis or parallel to x axis is 0°. The inclination of a vertical line (coinciding with y axis or parallel to y axis) is 90°.

- If θ is the inclination of a line l, then
  Gradient of line l = Slope$(m) = \tan \theta$, where $\theta \neq 90°$
- Slope of x-axis is zero and slope of y-axis is not defined.

Slope of a Line when Coordinates of Any Two Points on the Line are Given

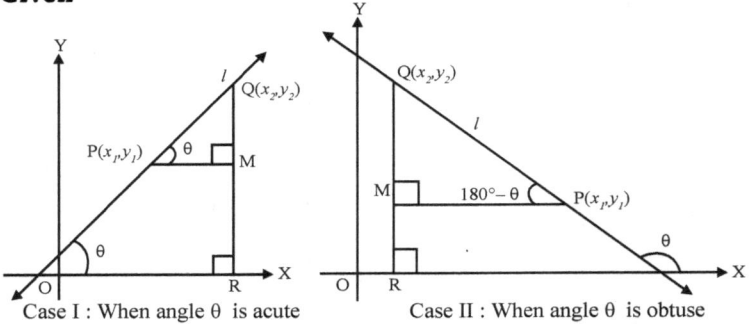

Case I : When angle θ is acute   Case II : When angle θ is obtuse

In both the cases(the angle is acute and obtuse) the slope m of the line l through the points (x_1, y_1) and (x_2, y_2) is given by:

$$m = \frac{y_2 - y_1}{x_2 - x_1} \text{ where } x_1 \neq x_2$$

Condition for Lines to be Parallel

Two non vertical lines l_1 and l_2 are parallel if and only if their slopes m_1 and m_2 are equal.

$$\text{or } \tan \alpha = \tan \beta$$

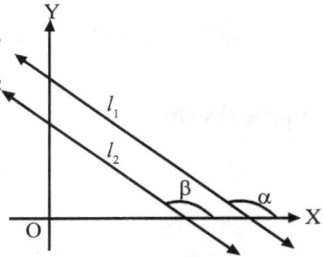

Condition for Lines to be Perpendicular

Two non vertical lines l_1 and l_2 are perpendicular to each other if and only if their slopes m_1 and m_2 are negative reciprocals of each other.

$$m_2 = -\frac{1}{m_1} \text{ or, } m_1 m_2 = -1$$

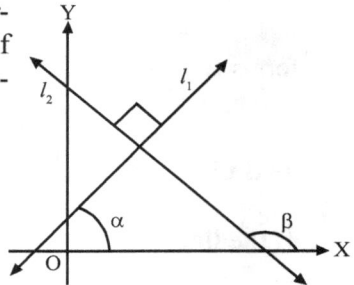

Angle Between Two Lines

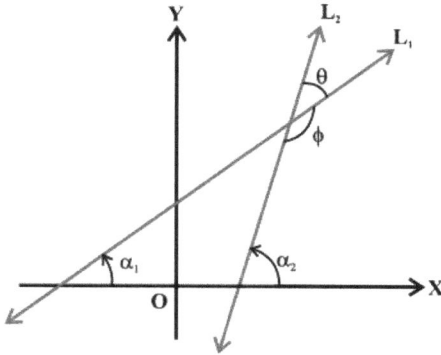

If θ be the acute angle between two lines L_1 and L_2 with slopes m_1 and m_2 respectively, then angle between the lines is given by

$$\tan\theta = \left| \frac{m_2 - m_1}{1 + m_2 m_1} \right|, \text{ where } 1 + m_1 m_2 \neq 0$$

The obtuse angle $\varphi = 180° - \theta$

Collinearity of Three Points

Three points A, B and C are collinear if and only if
Slope of AB = Slope of BC

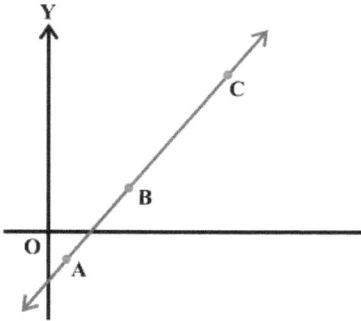

Equation of Vertical Line

The equation of a vertical line at a distance a is given by either $x = a$ or $x = -a$

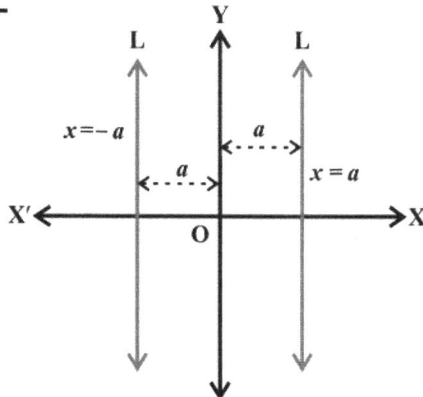

Equation of Horizontal Line

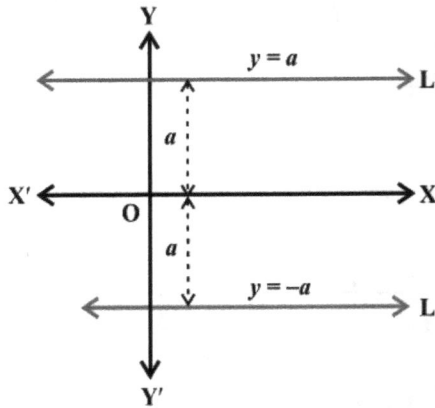

The equation of a horizontal line at a distance a is given by either $y = a$ or $y = -a$.

Point Slope Form

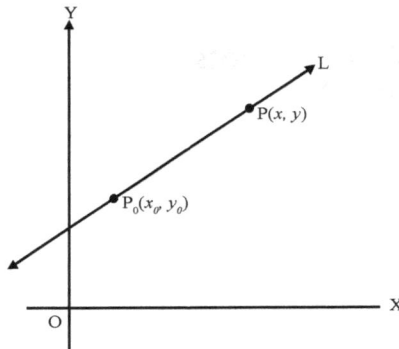

The point (x, y) lies on the line L with slope m through the fixed point (x_0, y_0), if and only if, its coordinates satisfy the equation

$$y - y_0 = m(x - x_0)$$

Two Point Form

Equation of the line passing through points (x_1, y_1) and (x_2, y_2) is given by

$$y - y_1 = \frac{y_2 - y_1}{x_2 - x_1}(x - x_1)$$

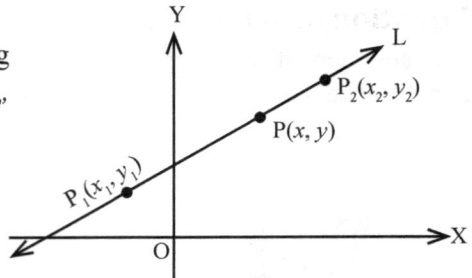

Slope Intercept Form

The point (x, y) on the line with slope m and x-intercept d lies on the line if and only if $y = m(x - d)$.

The point (x, y) on the line with slope m and y-intercept c lies on the line if and only if $y = mx + c$ (c is positive or negative depending on the direction of the intercept i.e positive or negative side of the y axis).

Intercept Form

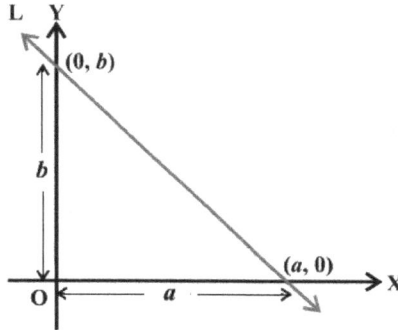

Equation of a line making intercepts a and b on the x axis and y axis respectively is given by

$$\frac{x}{a} + \frac{y}{b} = 1$$

Normal Form

Let the normal distance (OA) of line L from the origin be p and let the angle between the normal and the positive x axis be ω then the equation of the line is given by

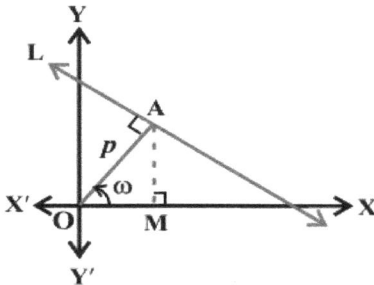

$$x \cos \omega + y \sin \omega = p$$

General Equation of a Line

Any equation of the form $Ax + By + C = 0$, where A and B are not zero simultaneously, is called the general equation of a line.

Different Forms of the Line $Ax + By + C = 0$

Slope Intercept Form

(i) If $B \neq 0$, $Ax + By + C = 0$ can be expressed as

$$y = -\frac{A}{B}x - \frac{C}{B} \text{ or } y = mx + c$$

where $m = -\frac{A}{B}$ and $c = -\frac{C}{B}$

(ii) If $B = 0$, then $x = -\frac{C}{A}$ which represents *a* vertical line with x

intercept $-\frac{C}{A}$ and undefined slope.

Intercept Form

(i) If $C \neq 0$, $Ax + By + C = 0$ can be expressed as

$$\frac{x}{-\dfrac{C}{A}} + \frac{y}{-\dfrac{C}{B}} = 1 \text{ or } \frac{x}{a} + \frac{y}{b} = 1$$

where $a = -\frac{C}{A}$ and $b = -\frac{C}{B}$

(ii) If $C = 0$, $Ax + By + C = 0$ reduces to $Ax + By = 0$. This line
has zero intercepts on the x axis and y axis, it passes through
the origin.

Normal Form

The normal form of the line $Ax + By + C = 0$ is
$x \cos \omega + y \sin \omega = p$, where

$$\cos \omega = \pm \frac{A}{\sqrt{A^2 + B^2}}, \quad \sin \omega = \pm \frac{B}{\sqrt{A^2 + B^2}} \text{ and } p = \pm \frac{C}{\sqrt{A^2 + B^2}}$$

Distance of a Point From a Line

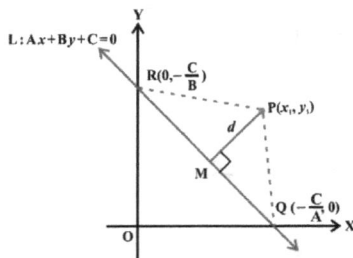

The perpendicular distance (d) of a line $Ax + By + C = 0$ from a point
$P(x_1, y_1)$ is given by

$$d = \frac{|Ax_1 + By_1 + C|}{\sqrt{A^2 + B^2}}$$

Mathematics Formulae

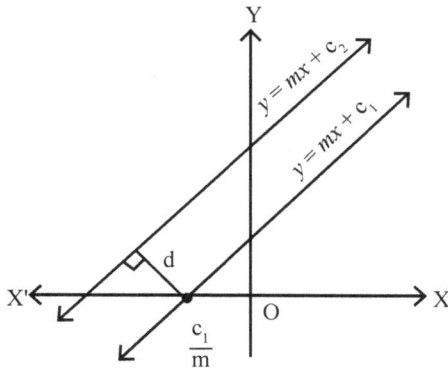

d) between two parallel lines $Ax \quad y + C_1$

$Ax \quad y + C_2$

$$d = \frac{|C_1 - C_2|}{\sqrt{ ^2 + ^2}}$$

CONIC SECTION

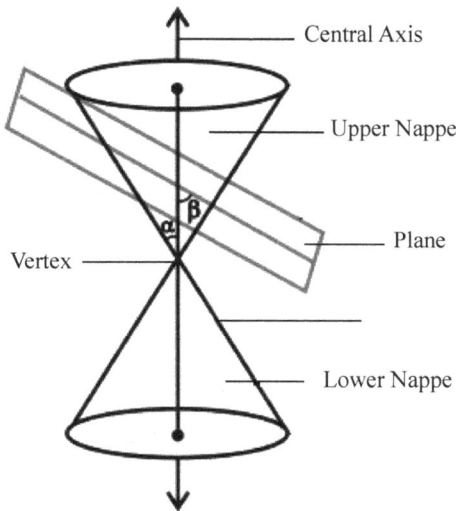

(i) *Conic Section* : The curve obtained by the intersection of a plane and a right circular cone is known as a conic section.

(ii)   : Two identical but opposite cones having a common vertex is known as a double napped cone.

(iii)   : The line (other than the central axis) joining the base of a cone to its vertex or apex is known as generator.

(iv) *Vertex*
     known as apex or vertex of the cone.

(v)   : The axis of symmetry of a right circular cone is known as central axis.

intersecting plane.

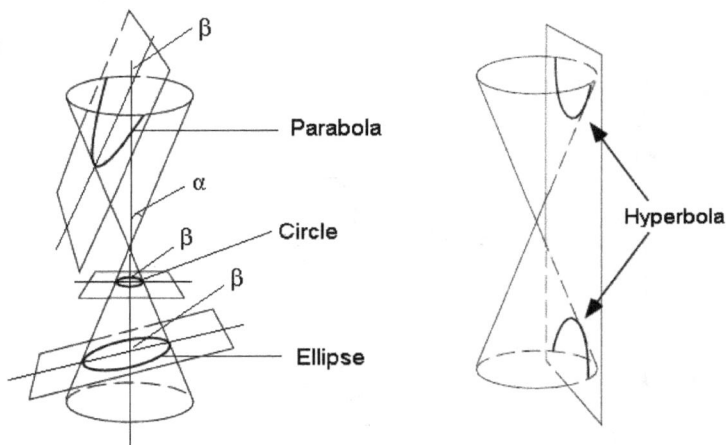

Parabola

Circle

Ellipse

Hyperbola

(i)   : If a plane is perpendicular to the central axis of the
           °, the section of the cone is known as a circle.

(ii)   : If a plane is not perpendicular to the central axis

     a parabola.

(iii)   : If a plane is not perpendicular to the central axis of
           °, the section of the cone is known
     as an ellipse.

(iv)   : If a plane intersects both the nappes of a cone

     hyperbola.

PARABOLA

Focus and Directrix : The set of all points in a plane that are equidis-

known as a parabola. The fixed point is called the focus and the fixed line is called the directrix.

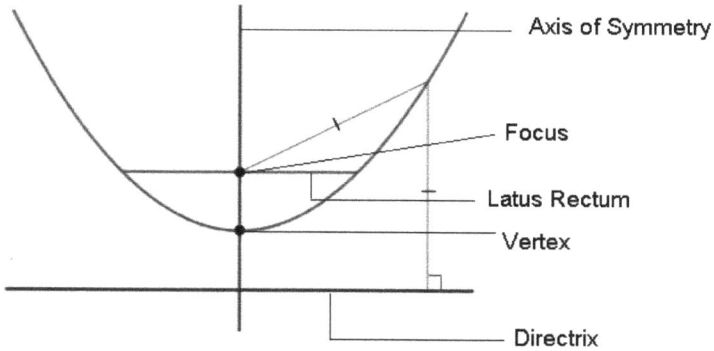

Axis : A line perpendicular to the directrix which passes through the focus is called the axis of the parabola.

Vertex : The point of intersection of parabola with the axis is known as the vertex of the parabola.

Latus Rectum : A line segment whose end points lie on the parabola and which is perpendicular to the axis of the parabola through the focus is known as the latus rectum of the parabola.

Different Orientations of a Parabola

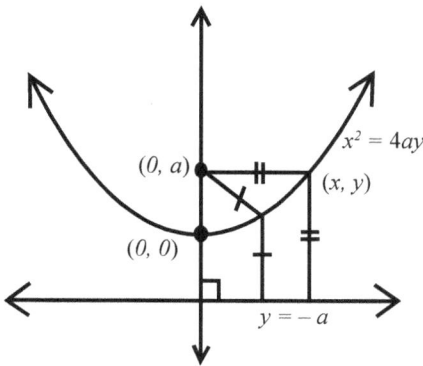

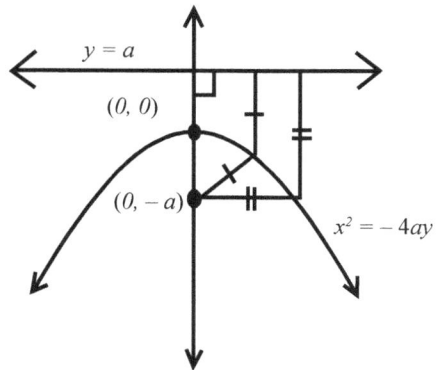

$x^2 = 4ax$

$x^2 = -4ax$

$x = -a$

$x = a$

$(0, 0)$ $(a, 0)$

$(-a, 0)$ $(0, 0)$

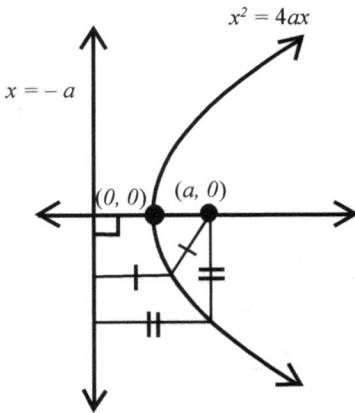

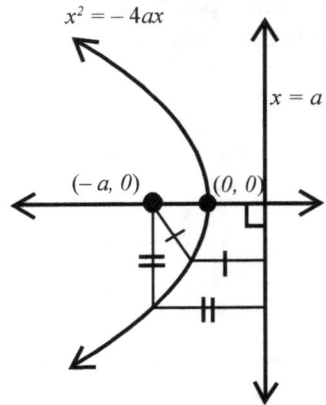

Properties of Parabola

Standard Equation	$x^2 = 4ay$ $(a > 0)$ Upward	$x^2 = -4ay$ $(a > 0)$ Downward	$y^2 = 4ax$ $(a > 0)$ Rightside	$y^2 = -4ax$ $(a > 0)$ Leftside
Directrix	$y = -a$	$y = a$	$x = -a$	$x = a$
Axis	$x = 0$	$x = 0$	$y = 0$	$y = 0$
Vertex	$(0,0)$	$(0,0)$	$(0,0)$	$(0,0)$
Focus	$(0,a)$	$(0, -a)$	$(a,0)$	$(-a,0)$
Focal distance of the point (x,y)	$a + y$	$a - y$	$a + x$	$a - x$
Tangent at the vertex	$y = 0$	$y = 0$	$x = 0$	$x = 0$
Length of latus rectum	4a	4a	4a	4a

ELLIPSE

An ellipse is the set of all points in a plane, the sum of whose distanc-

major axis.

$$P_1F + P_1F' = P_2F + P_2F' = P_3F + P_3F' = \text{constant} = 2a \, (> FF')$$

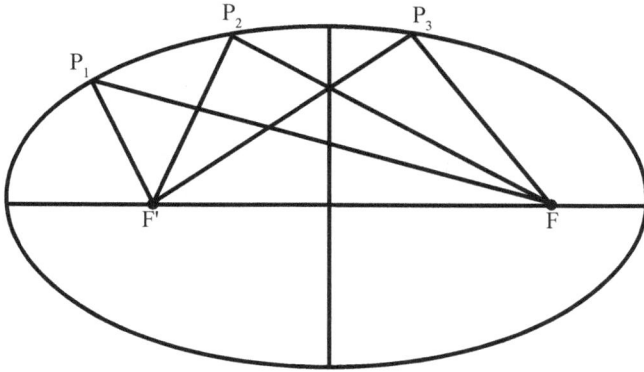

focus of an ellipse. In the above

Centre : The mid point of the line segment joining the two foci is known as the centre (O) of the ellipse.

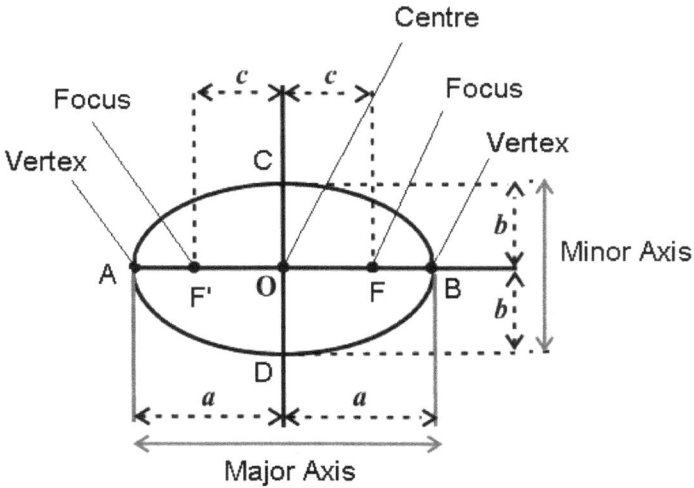

Major Axis : The line segment which passes through the two foci and whose end points lie on the ellipse is known as the major axis(AB). Length of the major axis is represented by *2a*.

Semi Major Axis: Half of major axis is known as semi major axis (AO or BO). Length of the semi major axis is represented by *a*.

Minor Axis : The line segment which passes through the centre and is perpendicular to the major axis is known as the minor axis (CD). Length of the minor axis is represented by *2b*.

Semi Minor Axis : Half of minor axis is known as semi minor axis (CO or DO). Length of the semi minor axis is represented by *b*.

Vertices : The end points of the major axis are known as the vertices of the ellipse. In the above figure points A and B represent the vertices.

Relationship between Semi-major Axis, Semi-minor Axis and the Distance of the Focus From the Centre of the Ellipse

If the length of the semi major axis, semi minor axis and the distance between the centre and the focus is *a, b* and *c* respectively, then

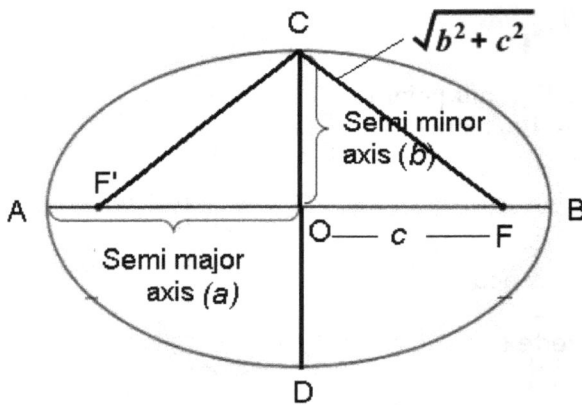

$$2\sqrt{b^2 + c^2} = 2a \text{ or } c = \sqrt{a^2 - b^2}$$

Special Cases

(i) If $c = 0$, *a* becomes equal to *b* and the ellipse reduces to a circle.

(ii) If $c = a$, then *b* becomes equal to 0 and the ellipse reduces to a line segment.

Eccentricity of an Ellipse

Eccentricity is a measure of how much the conic section deviates from being circular.

The eccentricity of an ellipse is the ratio of the distances from the centre of the ellipse to one of the foci and to one of the vertices of the ellipse. Eccentricity is represented by e and is given by $e = \dfrac{c}{a}$

Note:

For an ellipse $e < 1$, for a circle $e = 0$, for a parabola $e = 1$ and for hyperbola $e > 1$.

Standard Equation of an Ellipse

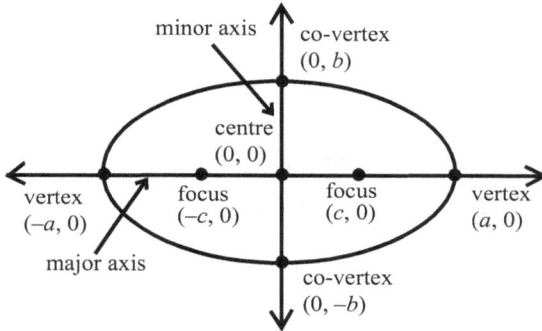

The equation of the ellipse with horizontal(along x axis) major axis and passing through the centre is given by $\dfrac{x^2}{a^2} + \dfrac{y^2}{b^2} = 1$

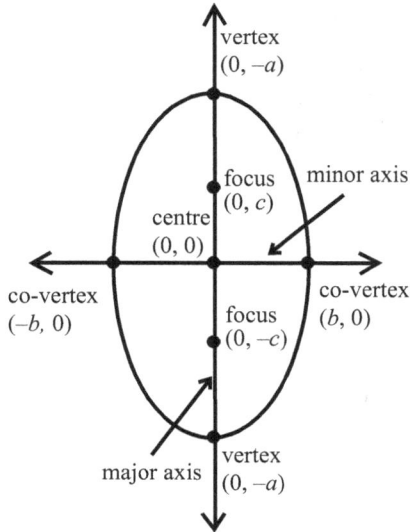

The equation of the ellipse with vertcal(along y axis) major axis and passing through the centre is given by $\dfrac{x^2}{b^2} + \dfrac{y^2}{a^2} = 1$

Latus Rectum

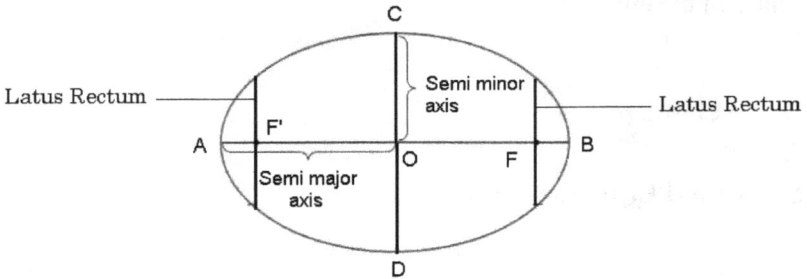

A line segment passing through any of the foci and perpendicular to the major axis is known as the latus rectum of an ellipse. The end points of the latus rectum lie on the ellipse.

Directrix and Focal Radius

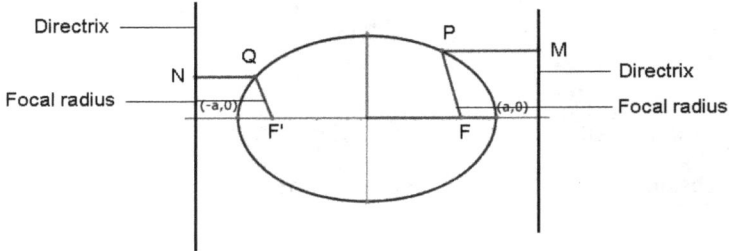

Directrix : It is a line parallel to the minor axis such that the distance from any point(P or Q) on the ellipse to the focus(F or F') is a constant fraction of that point's perpendicular distance (M or N) to the directrix, resulting in the equality

$$e = \frac{PF}{PM} \text{ or } e = \frac{QF'}{QN}$$

Focal Radius : The distance from a focus to a point on the ellipse is called focal radius (PF or QF').

Properties of Ellipse

1. Ellipse is symmetric with respect to both the coordinate axes.
2. The foci of an ellipse always lie on the major axis.
3. The sum of focal radii is constant (PF + PF' = 2a or QF + QF' = 2a)

Mathematics Formulae

Standard Equation	$\dfrac{x^2}{a^2}+\dfrac{y^2}{b^2}=1$ (Horizontal major axis)	$\dfrac{x^2}{b^2}+\dfrac{y^2}{a^2}=1$ (Vertical major axis)
Length of major axis	$2a$	$2a$
Length of minor axis	$2b$	$2b$
Equation of major axis	$y=0$	$x=0$
Equation of minor axis	$x=0$	$y=0$
Centre	$(0,0)$	$(0,0)$
Vertices	$(\pm a, 0)$	$(0, \pm a)$
Foci	$(\pm ae, 0)$	$(0, \pm ae)$
Distance between two foci	$2ae$	$2ae$
Eccentricity	$e=\dfrac{\sqrt{a^2-b^2}}{a}$	$e=\dfrac{\sqrt{a^2-b^2}}{a}$
Length of latus rectum	$\dfrac{2b^2}{a}$	$\dfrac{2b^2}{a}$
Equation of directrix	$x=\pm\dfrac{a}{e}$	$y=\pm\dfrac{a}{e}$
Distance between two directrix	$x=\dfrac{2a}{e}$	$x=\dfrac{2a}{e}$
Equation of tangent at the vertex	$x=\pm a$	$y=\pm a$

Parametric Coordinates

For the ellipse,

$$\frac{x^2}{a^2}+\frac{y^2}{b^2}=1 \ \text{ or } \ \frac{x^2}{b^2}+\frac{y^2}{a^2}=1$$

the parametric coordinates are given by $x = a\cos\theta$, $y = b\sin\theta$ where $0° \le \theta < 360°$

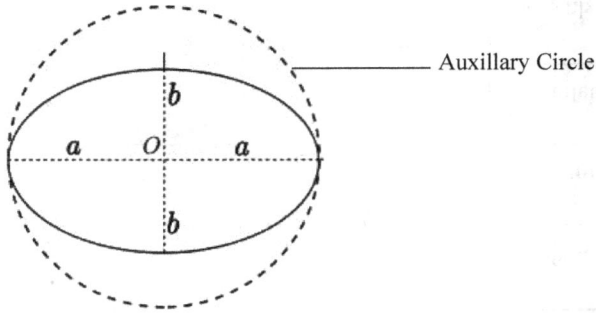

Auxillary Circle

The circle drawn with major axis as the diameter is known as an auxillary circle.

HYPERBOLA

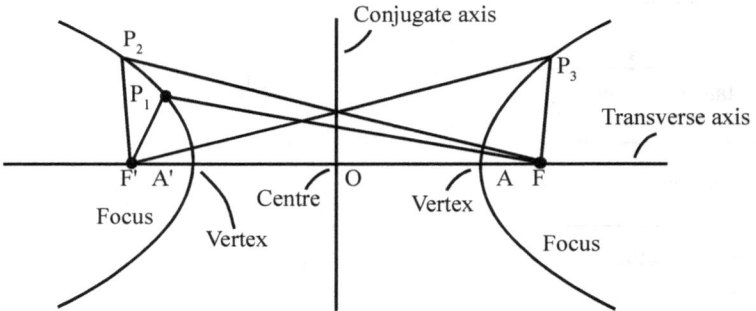

The set of all points in a plane, the difference of whose distances from

$$P_1F - P_1F' = P_2F - P_2F' = P_3F' - P_3F = \text{constant} = 2a$$

foci of the hyperbola.

Centre : The mid point of the line segment joining the two foci is known as the centre (O) of the hyperbola.

Transverse Axis : The line passing through the two foci is known as the transverse axis.

Conjugate Axis : The line which passes through the centre and is perpendicular to the transverse axis is known as the conjugate axis.

Vertex : The points at which the hyperbola intersects the transverse axis are known as the vertices(A and A') of the hyperbola.

Mathematics Formulae

Eccentricity

Like an ellipse, the eccentricity of the hyperbola is given by $e = \dfrac{c}{a}$

For a hyperbola, $e > 1$.

The foci are at a distance of ae from the centre in terms of eccentricity.

Standard Equation of Hyperbola

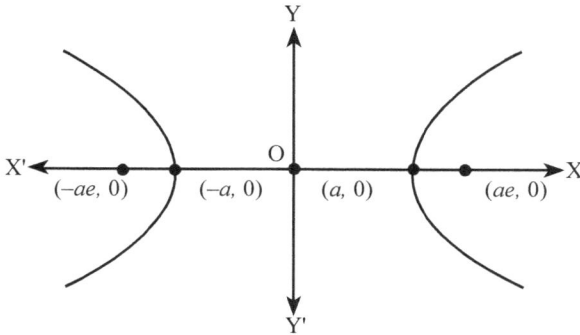

The equation of the hyperbola with focus on the x axis and passing through the centre is given by

$$\frac{x^2}{a^2} - \frac{y^2}{b^2} = 1$$

The equation of the hyperbola with focus on the y axis and passing through the centre is given by

$$\frac{x^2}{a^2} - \frac{y^2}{b^2} = -1$$

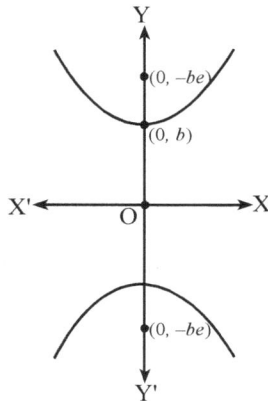

Equilateral Hyperbola : A hyperbola in which $a = b$ is known as an equilateral hyperbola.

Latus Rectum

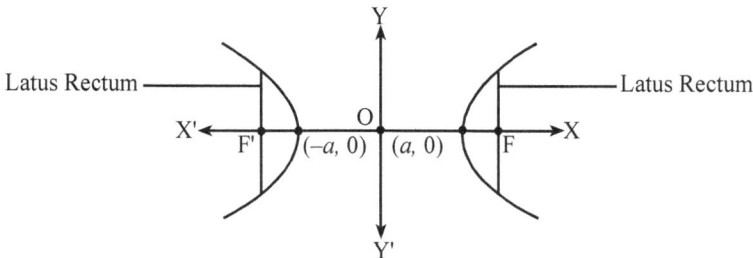

A line segment passing through any of the foci and perpendicular to the transverse axis is known as the latus rectum of a hyperbola. The end points of the latus rectum lie on the hyperbola.

Directrix

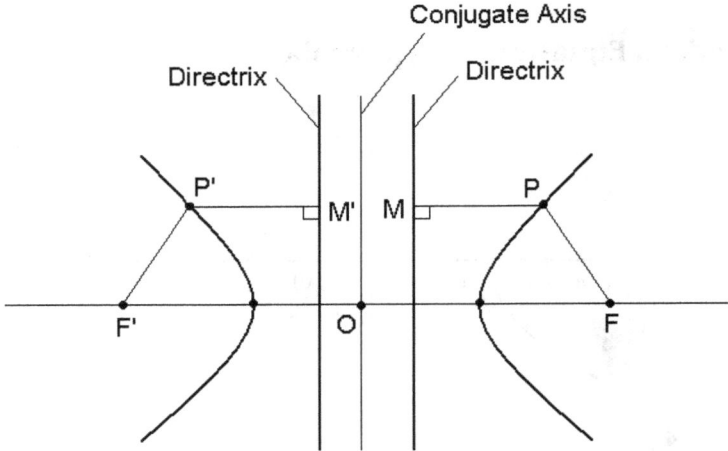

Directrix is a line parallel to the conjugate axis such that the distance from any point(P or P') on the hyperbola to the focus(F or F') is a constant fraction of that point's perpendicular distance (M or M') to the directrix, resulting in the equality

$$e = \frac{PF}{PM} \text{ or } e = \frac{P'F'}{P'M'}$$

Properties of Hyperbola

1. Hyperbola is symmetric with respect to both the axes.
2. The foci are always on the transverse axis.

	Hyperbola (Focus on x axis)	Conjugate Hyperbola (Focus on y axis)
Standard Equation	$\dfrac{x^2}{a^2} - \dfrac{y^2}{b^2} = 1$	$\dfrac{x^2}{a^2} - \dfrac{y^2}{b^2} = -1$
Length of transverse axis	$2a$	$2b$
Length of conjugate axis	$2b$	$2a$
Equation of transverse axis	$y = 0$	$x = 0$
Equation of conjugate axis	$x = 0$	$y = 0$

Centre		
Vertices		
Foci		
	2a	2b
	$e = \dfrac{\sqrt{^2 + ^2}}{a}$	$e = \dfrac{\sqrt{^2 + ^2}}{a}$
Length of latus rectum	$\dfrac{2^2}{a}$	$\dfrac{2a^2}{}$
	$x = \pm\dfrac{a}{e}$	$y = \pm\dfrac{}{e}$
	$x = \pm a$	$y = \pm b$

(i) For the hyperbola, $\dfrac{x^2}{2} - \dfrac{y^2}{2} = 1$

the parametric coordinates are given by   ,

(ii) For the hyperbola, $\dfrac{x^2}{2} - \dfrac{y^2}{2} = -1$

the parametric coordinates are given by   ,

CIRCLE

plane is called a circle.

If P( ) is any point on a circle with centre C( ) and radius r then the equation of the circle is given by
$$(x - h)^2 + (y - k)^2 = r^2$$

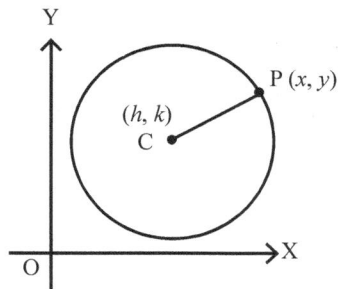

If P( ) is any point on a circle with centre at the origin and radius r then the equation of the circle is given by
$$x^2 + y^2 = r^2$$

General Equation of a Circle

The equation of a circle with centre $(-g, -f)$ and radius $\sqrt{g^2 + f^2 - c}$ is given by $x^2 + y^2 + 2gx + 2fy + c = 0$ where g, f and c are constants.

Conditions for an Equation to represent a Circle

A general equation of second degree
$ax^2 + 2hxy + by^2 + 2gx + 2fy + c = 0$ in x, y represents a circle if
(i) $2h = 0$ (Coefficient of $xy = 0$)
(ii) $a = b$ (Coefficient of $x^2 = y^2$)

Nature of Circle

(i) If $g^2 + f^2 - c > 0$, then the general equation represents real circle with centre at $(-g, -f)$.
(ii) If $g^2 + f^2 - c = 0$, then the general equation represents a point circle (radius zero).
(iii) If $g^2 + f^2 - c < 0$, then the general equation represents an imaginary circle (centre is real but radius is imaginary).

Different Forms of Equation of a Circle
Circle Touching the x Axis

The equation of the circle touching the x axis and with centre $C(h, k)$ is given by

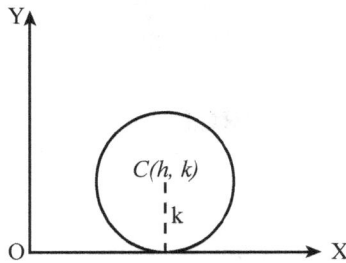

$$(x - h)^2 + (y - k)^2 = k^2$$

Circle Touching the y Axis

The equation of the circle touching the y axis and with centre $C(h, k)$ is given by

$$(x - h)^2 + (y - k)^2 = h^2$$

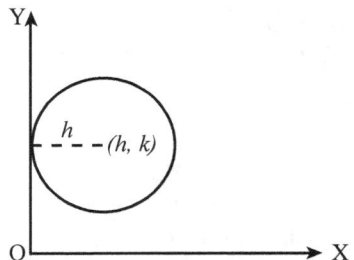

Circle Touching Both x and y Axis

The equation of the circle touching both the coordinate axis and having radius g is given by

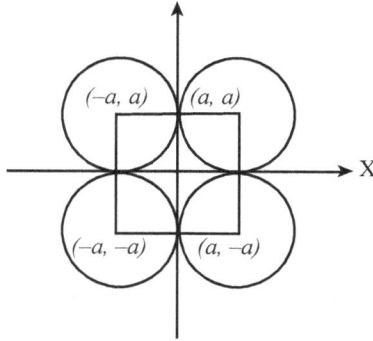

$$(x \pm a)^2 + (y \pm a)^2 = a^2$$

Equation of a Circle in Diametric Form

If $A(x_1, y_1)$ and $B(x_2, y_2)$ are the end points of a diameter, then the equation of the circle is given by

$$(x - x_1)(x - x_2) + (y - y_1)(y - y_2) = 0$$

$$\text{Centre} = \left(\frac{x_1 + x_2}{2}, \frac{y_1 + y_2}{2} \right)$$

$$\text{Radius} = \sqrt{\left(\frac{x_1 - x_2}{2} \right)^2 + \left(\frac{y_1 - y_2}{2} \right)^2}$$

Intercepts Made by a Circle on the Coordinate Axes

(i) Intercepts are always positive.

(ii) The length of the intercept made by the circle
$x^2 + y^2 + 2gx + 2fy + c = 0$ on

x axis $= 2\sqrt{g^2 - c}$ and y axis $= 2\sqrt{f^2 - c}$

(iii) If the circle touches x axis, then $c = g^2$

(iv) If the circle touches y axis, then $c = f^2$

(v) If the circle touches both the coordinate axes, then $c = g^2 = f^2$

Parametric Equation of a Circle

Let $P(x, y)$ be any point on the circle with centre at the origin and radius a. Let OP make an angle θ with the x axis, then

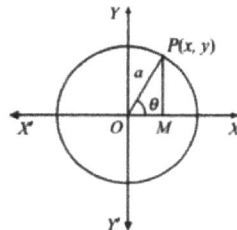

(i) the parametric equation of the circle $x^2 + y^2 = a^2$ is
$x = aCos\ \theta$,
$y = aSin\ \theta$, where $0° \leq \theta \leq 360°$

Note: The parametric equation of the circle
$(x - h)^2 + (y - k)^2 = r^2$ is $x = h + rCos\ \theta$ and $y = k + rSin\ \theta$

Position of a point with respect to a circle

Let $P(x_1, y_1)$ be a point on the circle
$x^2 + y^2 + 2gx + 2fy + c = 0$, then
  (i) the point lies on the circle if $x_1^2 + y_1^2 + 2gx_1 + 2fy_1 + c = 0$
  (ii) the point lies outside the circle if $x_1^2 + y_1^2 + 2gx_1 + 2fy_1 + c > 0$
  (iii) the point lies inside the circle if $x_1^2 + y_1^2 + 2gx_1 + 2fy_1 + c < 0$

Equation of a Circle through Three non Collinear Points

If $A(x_1, y_1)$, $B(x_2, y_2)$ and $C(x_3, y_3)$ are three non collinear points, then the equation of the circle through these three points is given by

$$\begin{vmatrix} x^2 + y^2 & x & y & 1 \\ x_1^2 + y_1^2 & x_1 & y_1 & 1 \\ x_2^2 + y_2^2 & x_2 & y_2 & 1 \\ x_3^2 + y_3^2 & x_3 & y_3 & 1 \end{vmatrix} = 0$$

Contact between Two Circles

If $A(x_1, y_1)$ and $B(x_2, y_2)$ be the centre of two circles with radii r_1 and r_2 respectively, then –
  (i) The circles will intersect at two real and distinct points if and only if
  $|r_1 - r_2| < AB < r_1 + r_2$

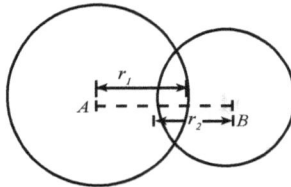

  (ii) The circles will touch each other internally if and only if
  $AB = |r_1 - r_2|$ and

  Point of contact (C) $= \left(\dfrac{r_1 x_2 - r_2 x_1}{r_1 - r_2}, \dfrac{r_1 y_2 - r_2 y_1}{r_1 - r_2} \right)$

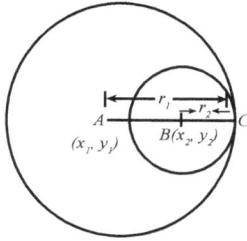

(iii) The circles will touch each other externally if and only if
$AB = r_1 + r_2$ and

Point of contact (C) = $\left(\dfrac{r_1 x_2 + r_2 x_1}{r_1 + r_2}, \dfrac{r_1 y_2 + r_2 y_1}{r_1 + r_2} \right)$

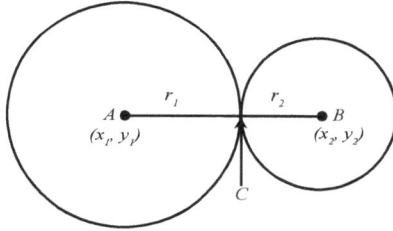

(iv) One circle is contained in the other if $AB < |r_1 - r_2|$.

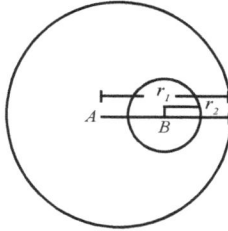

(v) One circle is outside the other circle if $AB > r_1 + r_2$

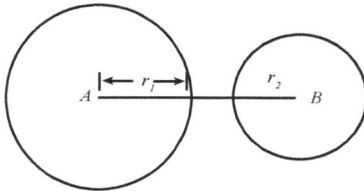

Equations of Tangent

(i) The equation of a tangent at the point $P(x_1, y_1)$ to the circle $x^2 + y^2 = r^2$ is given by $xx_1 + yy_1 = r^2$

(ii) The equation of a tangent at the point $P(x_1, y_1)$ to the circle $x^2 + y^2 + 2gx + 2fy + c = 0$ is given by
$xx_1 + yy_1 + g(x + x_1) + f(y + y_1) + c = 0$

(iii) The equation of a tangent to the circle $x^2 + y^2 = r^2$ with slope m

is $y = mx \pm r\sqrt{1 + m^2}$

Coordinates of the point of contact $= \left(\pm\dfrac{rm}{\sqrt{1+m^2}}, \pm\dfrac{r}{\sqrt{1+m^2}} \right)$

Condition of Tangent

- A line will be a tangent to the circle if and only if the perpendicular distance from the centre of the circle to the line is equal to the radius of the circle.

- The straight line $y = mx + c$ will be a tangent to the circle $x^2 + y^2 = r^2$ if $c = \pm r\sqrt{1 + m^2}$

Length of Tangent

Let $P(x_1, y_1)$ be a point outside the circle
$x^2 + y^2 + 2gx + 2fy + c = 0$ then,
Length of tangent $= \sqrt{x_1^2 + y_1^2 + 2gx_1 + 2fy_1 + c}$

Equation of Pair of Tangent

Let $P(x_1, y_1)$ be a point outside the circle

$x^2 + y^2 + 2gx + 2fy + c = 0$
then the equation of the pair of tangent is $SS_1 = T^2$, where

$S = x^2 + y^2 + 2gx + 2fy + c$

$S_1 = x_1^2 + y_1^2 + 2gx_1 + 2fy_1 + c$

$T = xx_1 + yy_1 + g(x + x_1) + f^2(y + y_1) + c$

Note: The pair of tangents to the circle $x^2 + y^2 + 2gx + 2fy + c = 0$ from the origin are at right angles if $g^2 + f^2 = 2c$

Angle of Intersection of Two Circles

The angle between two circles is the angle between their tangents at their point of intersection.

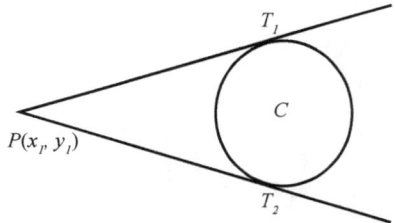

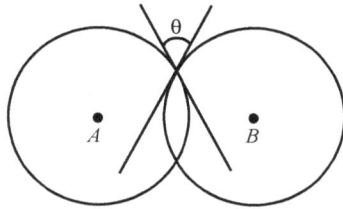

The angle θ between two circles $x^2 + y^2 + 2g_1x + 2f_1y + c_1$ and $x^2 + y^2 + 2g_2x + 2f_2y + c_2$ is given by

$$\cos\theta = \pm\frac{2g_1g_2 + 2f_1f_2 - c_1 - c_2}{2\sqrt{g_1^2 + f_1^2 - c_1} \cdot \sqrt{g_2^2 + f_2^2 - c_2}}$$

Orthogonal Intersection of Circles

When two circles intersect at right angles, they are said to intersect orthogonally.

The condition for the two circles $x^2 + y^2 + 2g_1x + 2f_1y + c_1$ and $x^2 + y^2 + 2g_2x + 2f_2y + c_2$ to intersect orthogonally is given by $2g_1g_2 + 2f_1f_2 = c_1 + c_2$

Equation of a Circle through Two given points

The equation of the circle passing through two given points $A(x_1, y_1)$ and $B(x_2, y_2)$ is given by

$$(x - x_1)(x - x_1) + (y - y_1)(y - y_2) + k \begin{vmatrix} x & y & 1 \\ x_1 & y_1 & 1 \\ x_2 & y_2 & 1 \end{vmatrix} = 0$$

where $k \in R$

Common Tangents of a Circle

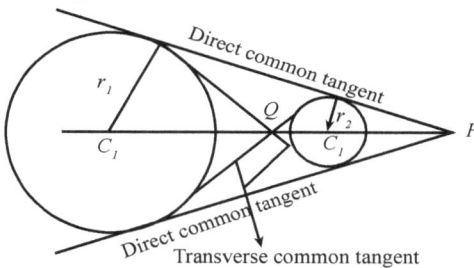

Direct Common Tangent

The direct common tangent of two circles meet at a point (P) which lies on the line (C_1C_2) joining the centres of the two circles and divide the line joining the two centres externally in the ratio of their radii (r_1, r_2).

Transverse Common Tangent

The transverse common tangent of two circles meet at a point (Q) which lies on the line (C_1C_2) joining the centres of the two circles and divide the line joining the two centres internally in the ratio of their radii (r_1, r_2).

THREE DIMENSIONAL COORDINATE GEOMETRY

Coordinate Axes

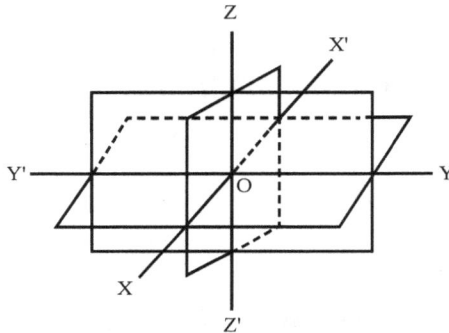

XOX' is called the x axis, YOY' is called the y axis and ZOZ' is called the z axis. The three axis are perpendicular to each other. The three axis together are called coordinate axes.

Coordinate Plane

The planes XOY, YOZ and ZOX are known as XY-plane, YZ-plane and ZX-plane respectively.

The point O is the origin of the coordinate system.

Octants

The XY-plane, YZ-plane and ZX-plane divide the space into eight

represented by I, II, III, IV, V, VI, VII and VIII respectively.

Let P be any point in space. If we draw perpendicular PM on the XY plane and ML on the x axis then the coordinates of the point P is given by ( ) where OL$= x$, ML $= y$ and PM $= z$.

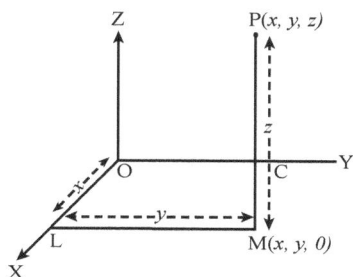

- The coordinates of the origin $= (0,0,0)$
- The coordinates of any point on the x axis $= (x,0,0)$
- The coordinates of any point on the y axis $= (0,y,0)$
- The coordinates of any point on the z axis $= (0,0,z)$

Signs of Coordinates in Various Octants

Octants→ Co-ordinates↓	I	II	III	IV	V	VI	VII	VIII
x	+	−	−	+	+	−	−	+
y	+	+	−	−	+	+	−	−
z	+	+	+	+	−	−	−	−

Distance Formula

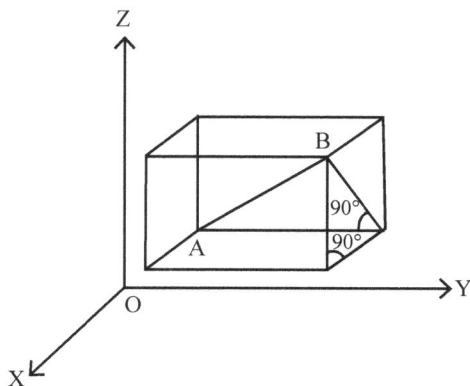

The distance between two points $A\,(x_1, y_1, z_1)$ and $B(x_2, y_2, z_2)$ is given by

$$AB = \sqrt{(x_2 - x_1)^2 + (y_2 - y_1)^2 + (z_2 - z_1)^2}$$

The distance of a point from the origin is given by $\sqrt{x_2^2 + y_2^2 + z_2^2}$

(i) The coordinates of the point which divides the line segment joining two points A $(x_1, y_1, z_1$ $x_2, y_2, z_2)$ internally in the ratio $m : n$ is given by

$$\left(\frac{mx_2 + nx_1}{m+n}, \frac{my_2 + ny_1}{m+n}, \frac{mz_2 + nz_1}{m+n} \right)$$

(ii) The coordinates of the point which divides the line segment joining two points A $(x_1, y_1, z_1$ $x_2, y_2, z_2)$ externally in the ratio $m : n$ is given by

$$\left(\frac{mx_2 - nx_1}{m-n}, \frac{my_2 - ny_1}{m-n}, \frac{mz_2 - nz_1}{m-n} \right)$$

(i) The coordinates of the mid point of the line segment joining two points A $(x_1, y_1, z_1$ $x_2, y_2, z_2)$ is

$$\left(\frac{x_1 + x_2}{2}, \frac{y_1 + y_2}{2}, \frac{z_1 + z_2}{2} \right)$$

(ii) The coordinates of the point which divides the line segment joining two points A $(x_1, y_1, z_1$ $x_2, y_2, z_2)$ in the ratio $k{:}1$ is given by

$$\left(\frac{kx_2 + x_1}{1+k}, \frac{ky_2 + y_1}{1+k}, \frac{kz_2 + z_1}{1+k} \right)$$

The coordinates of the centroid of a triangle with vertices A $(x_1, y_1, z_1$), $x_2, y_2, z_2)$ and C $(x_3, y_3, z_3$) is given by

$$\left(\frac{x_1 + x_2 + x_3}{3}, \frac{y_1 + y_2 + y_3}{3}, \frac{z_1 + z_2 + z_3}{3} \right)$$

LINE IN SPACE

If a directed line L passing through the origin
and z axes
respectively, then

tion angles.

tion cosines of the directed line L.

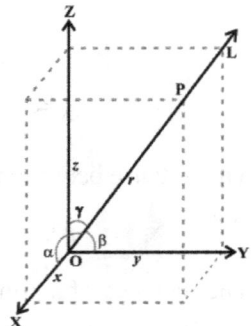

Mathematics Formulae

(iii) The direction cosines are generally represented by l, m and n i.e.
$l = \cos \alpha$, $m = \cos \beta$ and $n = \cos \gamma$

Direction Ratio

Any three numbers a, b, c which are proportional to the direction cosines l, m, n of a line are known as the direction ratios of the line.

(i) $\dfrac{l}{a} = \dfrac{m}{b} = \dfrac{n}{c} = k$ $k \neq 0$, $k = $ constant

(ii) $l = \pm\dfrac{a}{\sqrt{a^2 + b^2 + c^2}}$, $m = \pm\dfrac{b}{\sqrt{a^2 + b^2 + c^2}}$, $n = \pm\dfrac{c}{\sqrt{a^2 + b^2 + c^2}}$

Relation Between the Direction Cosines of a Line

If l, m, n are the direction cosines of a line, then $l^2 + m^2 + n^2 = 1$

Direction Cosines of a Line Passing Through Two Points

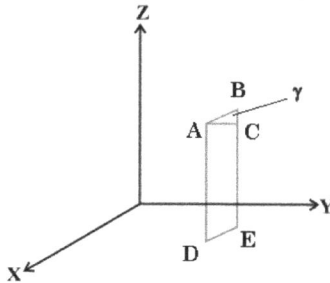

The direction cosines of the line segment joining the points

$A\,(x_1, y_1, z_1)$ and $B(x_2, y_2, z_2)$ are $\dfrac{x_2 - x_1}{AB}, \dfrac{y_2 - y_1}{AB}, \dfrac{z_2 - z_1}{AB}$

where $AB = \sqrt{(x_2 - x_1)^2 + (y_2 - y_1)^2 + (z_2 - z_1)^2}$

Equation of a Line

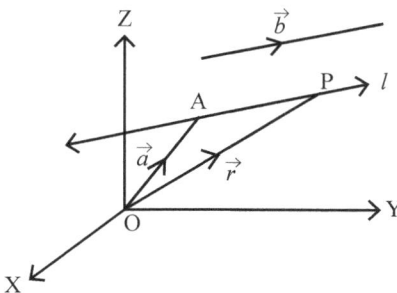

Vector Equation

The vector equation of the line l which is parallel to vector b and passes through point A is given by

$$\vec{r} = \vec{a} + \lambda \vec{b}$$

where $\vec{r}$ is the position vector of an arbitray point P, $\vec{a}$ is the position vector of the given point A with respect to origin and λ is a real number.

Cartesian Equation

The Cartesian equation of the line that passes through the point (x_1, y_1, z_1) with direction ratios a, b, c is given by

$$\frac{x - x_1}{a} = \frac{y - y_1}{b} = \frac{z - z_1}{c}$$

If l, m, n are the direction cosines, then

$$\frac{x - x_1}{l} = \frac{y - y_1}{m} = \frac{z - z_1}{n}$$

Equation of a Line Passing Through Two Points

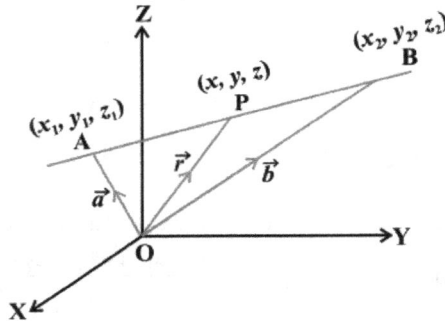

Vector Equation

If vector a and vector b are the position vectors of the points A (x_1, y_1, z_1) and B(x_2, y_2, z_2) respectively and vector r be the position vector of an arbitrary point P(x, y, z), then the vector equation is given by

$$\vec{r} = \vec{a} + \lambda(\vec{b} - \vec{a}), \text{ where } \lambda \in R$$

Cartesian Equation

The cartesian equation of the line joining two points A(x_1, y_1, z_1) and B(x_2, y_2, z_2) is given by

$$\frac{x - x_1}{x_2 - x_1} = \frac{y - y_1}{y_2 - y_1} = \frac{z - z_1}{z_2 - z_1}$$

Mathematics Formulae

Angle Between Two Lines

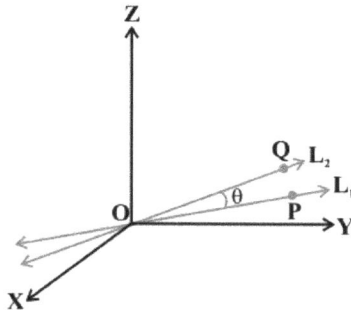

- The angle θ between two lines L_1 and L_2 passing through the origin and with direction ratios a_1, b_1, c_1 and a_2, b_2, c_2 respectively is given by

$$\cos\theta = \left| \frac{a_1 a_2 + b_1 b_2 + c_1 c_2}{\sqrt{a_1^2 + b_1^2 + c_1^2}\sqrt{a_2^2 + b_2^2 + c_2^2}} \right|$$

- If l_1, m_1, n_1 and l_2, m_2, n_2 be the direction cosines of two lines L_1 and L_2 respectively, then the angle θ between the lines is given by

$$\cos\theta = \left| l_1 l_2 + m_1 m_2 + n_1 n_2 \right|$$

(i) Two lines with direction ratios a_1, b_1, c_1 and a_2, b_2, c_2 are perpendicular if $\theta = 90°$ or $a_1 a_2 + b_1 b_2 + c_1 c_2 = 0$.

(ii) Two lines with direction ratios a_1, b_1, c_1 and a_2, b_2, c_2 are parallel if $\theta = 0°$ or $\dfrac{a_1}{a_2} = \dfrac{b_1}{b_2} = \dfrac{c_1}{c_2}$

Shortest Distance between Two Lines

In three dimensional coordinate system,

(i) the shortest distance between two intersecting lines is zero.

(ii) the shortest distance between two parallel lines is the perpendicular distance between them.

(iii) For skew lines the shortest distance is perpendicular to both the lines.

In space the lines which are neither parallel nor intersecting are known as *skew lines*. They lie in different planes.

Distance between Two Skew Lines

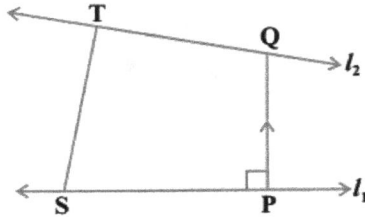

Vector Form

The shortest distance between two skew lines l_1 and l_2 with equations $\vec{r} = \vec{a_1} + \lambda \vec{b_1}$ and $\vec{r} = \vec{a_2} + \mu \vec{b_2}$ respectively is given by

$$d = \left| \frac{(\vec{b_1} \times \vec{b_2}) \cdot (\vec{a_2} - \vec{a_1})}{|\vec{b_1} \times \vec{b_2}|} \right|$$

Cartesian Form

The shortest distance between two skew lines l_1 and l_2 with equations

$$l_1 : \frac{x - x_1}{a_1} = \frac{y - y_1}{b_1} = \frac{z - z_1}{c_1} \text{ and } l_2 : \frac{x - x_2}{a_2} = \frac{y - y_2}{b_2} = \frac{z - z_2}{c_2} \text{ is given by}$$

$$\frac{\begin{vmatrix} x_2 - x_1 & y_2 - y_1 & z_2 - z_1 \\ a_1 & b_1 & c_1 \\ a_2 & b_2 & c_2 \end{vmatrix}}{\sqrt{(b_1 c_2 - b_2 c_1)^2 + (c_1 a_2 - c_2 a_1)^2 + (a_1 b_2 - a_2 b_1)^2}}$$

Distance Between Parallel Lines

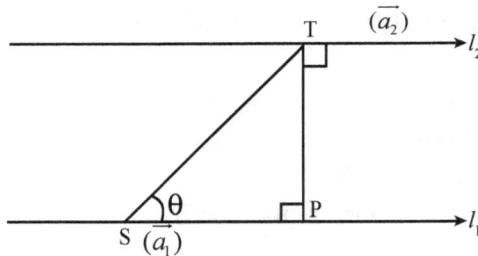

The distance between two parallel lines l_1 and l_2 with equations $\vec{r} = \vec{a_1} + \lambda \vec{b}$ and $\vec{r} = \vec{a_2} + \mu \vec{b}$ is given by

$$d = |\overline{PT}| = \left| \frac{\vec{b} \times (\vec{a_2} - \vec{a_1})}{|\vec{b}|} \right|$$

PLANE

A plane is determined uniquely if any one of the following is known:
(i) The equation of a plane in normal form.
(ii) The equation of a plane passes through a given point and perpendicular to a given vector.
(iii) The equation of the plane passes through three non collinear points.

Vector Form

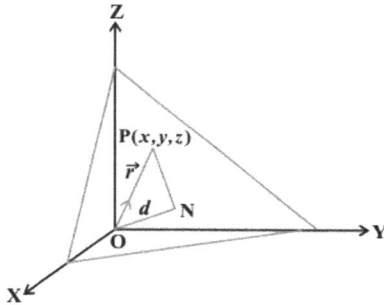

If vector r is the position vector of the point P(   ),   is the perpendicular distance of the plane from the origin and $\hat{n}$ the unit normal vector along $\overline{ON}$, then the equation of the plane is given by
$r \cdot \hat{n} = d$

Cartesian Form

If n are the direction cosines and   is the perpendicular distance of the plane from the origin, then equation of the plane is given by
$$+ my + nz = d$$

Vector Form

If vector r be the position vector of the point P(   ), vector a the position vector of the point Q through which the plane passes and vector N be perpendicular to the plane, then the equation of the plane is given by

$r - a$ $=$

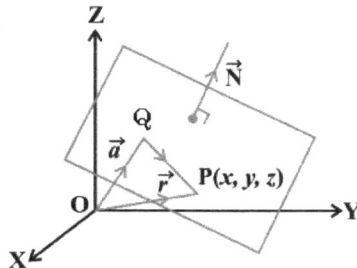

Cartesian Form

If A, B, C are the direction ratios of the vector N and the coordinates of P and Q be (x, y, z) and (x_1, y_1, z_1) respectively, then the equation of the plane is given by

$$A(x - x_1) + B(y - y_1) + C(z - z_1) = 0$$

Equation of the Plane through Three Non Collinear Points

Vector Form

If vector r be the position vector of the point $P(x, y, z)$, vector a, vector b and vector c be the position vectors of three non collinear points R, S and T respectively, then the equation of the plane is given by

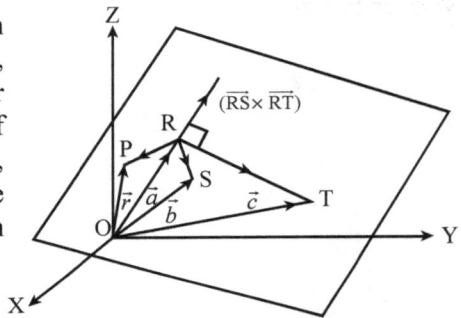

$$(\vec{r} - \vec{a}) \times [(\vec{b} - \vec{a}) \times (\vec{c} - \vec{a})] = 0$$

Cartesian Form

If vector r be the position vector of the point $P(x, y, z)$, (x_1, y_1, z_1), (x_2, y_2, z_2) and (x_3, y_3, z_3) be the coordinates of the non collinear points R, S and T respectively, then the equation of the plane is given by

$$\begin{vmatrix} x - x_1 & y - y_1 & z - z_1 \\ x_2 - x_1 & y_2 - y_1 & z_2 - z_1 \\ x_3 - x_1 & y_3 - y_1 & z_3 - z_1 \end{vmatrix} = 0$$

Intercept Form of the Equation of a Plane

The equation of the plane which makes intercepts a, b, c with x, y and z axis respectively is given by $\dfrac{x}{a} + \dfrac{y}{b} + \dfrac{z}{c} = 1$

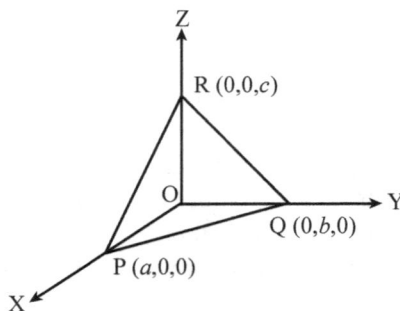

Plane Passing through the Intersection of Two Given Planes

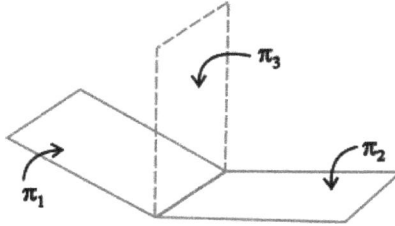

Vector Form

If two planes π_1 and π_2 have equations $\vec{r} \cdot \hat{n}_1 = d_1$ and $\vec{r} \cdot \hat{n}_2 = d_2$ respectively, then the equation of the plane (π_3) passing through the intersection of these two planes is given by $\vec{r} \cdot (\vec{n}_1 + \lambda \vec{n}_2) = d_1 + \lambda d_2$ where λ is a non zero constant.

Cartesian Form

The cartesian equation of the plane passing through the intersection of two planes is given by

$$(A_1 x + B_1 y + C_1 z - d_1) + \lambda(A_2 x + B_2 y + C_2 z - d_2) = 0$$

Coplanarity of Two Lines

Vector Form

Two lines $\vec{r} = \vec{a}_1 + \lambda \vec{b}_1$ and $\vec{r} = \vec{a}_2 + \mu \vec{b}_2$ are coplanar if and only if $(\vec{a}_2 - \vec{a}_1) \cdot (\vec{b}_1 \times \vec{b}_2) = 0$

Cartesian Form

If (x_1, y_1, z_1) and (x_2, y_2, z_2) be the coordinates of points A and B respectively and if a_1, b_1, c_1 and a_2, b_2, c_2 be the direction ratios of vector b_1 and vector b_2 respectively, then

$$\overline{AB} = (x_2 - x_1)\hat{i} + (y_2 - y_1)\hat{j} + (z_2 - z_1)\hat{k}$$
$$\vec{b}_1 = a_1\hat{i} + b_1\hat{j} + c_1\hat{k} \text{ and } \vec{b}_2 = a_2\hat{i} + b_2\hat{j} + c_2\hat{k}$$

The given lines are coplanar if

$$\begin{vmatrix} x_2 - x_1 & y_2 - y_1 & z_2 - z_1 \\ a_1 & b_1 & c_1 \\ a_2 & b_2 & c_2 \end{vmatrix} = 0$$

Angle between Two Planes

The angle between two planes is defined as the angle between their normals.

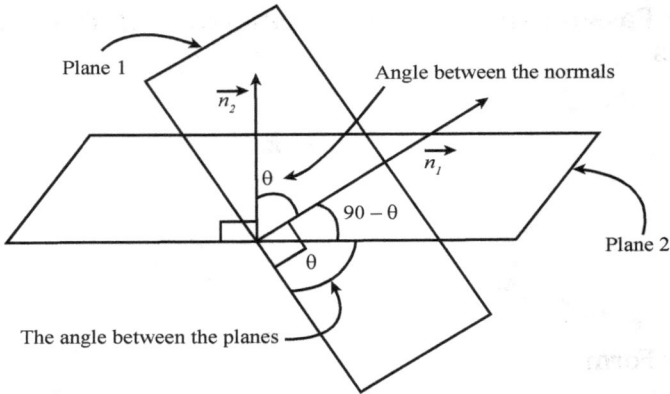

Plane 1

Angle between the normals

$\vec{n_2}$

$\vec{n_1}$

θ

$90 - \theta$

Plane 2

θ

The angle between the planes

Vector Form

The angle θ between two planes with normals as vector n_1 and vector n_2 respectively is given by

$$\cos\theta = \left| \frac{\vec{n_1} \cdot \vec{n_2}}{|\vec{n_1}| |\vec{n_2}|} \right|$$

Cartesian Form

The angle θ between two planes,
$A_1 x + B_1 y + C_1 z + D_1 = 0$ and
$A_2 x + B_2 y + C_2 z + D_2 = 0$
is given by

$$\cos\theta = \left| \frac{A_1 A_2 + B_1 B_2 + C_1 C_2}{\sqrt{A_1^2 + B_1^2 + C_1^2} \sqrt{A_2^2 + B_2^2 + C_2^2}} \right|$$

where A_1, B_1, C_1 and A_2, B_2, C_2 are the direction ratios of the normal to the planes respectively.

Note:

(i) If the planes are at right angles, then
$\cos\theta = A_1 A_2 + B_1 B_2 + C_1 C_2 = 0$

(ii) If the planes are parallel, then $\dfrac{A_1}{A_2} = \dfrac{B_1}{B_2} = \dfrac{C_1}{C_2}$

Distance of a Point from a Plane

Vector Form

Let P be a point in plane π_2 with position vector $\vec{a}$

The equation of the unit vector normal to π_2 is given by $\vec{r} \cdot \hat{n} = \vec{a} \cdot \hat{n}$

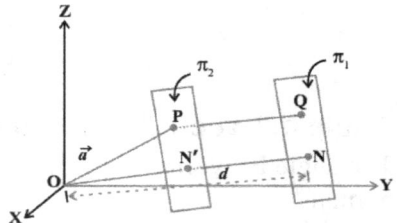

$_1$ is given by $|d - a \cdot \hat{n}|$

Cartesian Form

The distance between the point P( ) and the plane
$Ax + By + Cz + D = 0$ is given by

$$\left| \frac{x_1 \quad y_1 \quad z_1 -}{\sqrt{\quad 2 \quad 2 \quad 2}} \right|$$

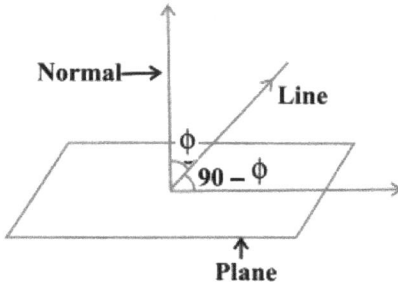

The angle between a line and a plane is the complement of the angle between the line and the normal to the plane.

The angle between the line = $+ \lambda$ and the plane $r \cdot n = d$ is given by

$$-\phi = \qquad \phi = \left| \frac{\cdot}{\| \cdot \| \cdot \| \cdot \|} \right|$$

SPHERE

called a sphere. It is a three dimensional shape. The shortest distance between any two points on a sphere is known as *geodesic*.

If P( ) is any point on a sphere with centre C( ) and radius r then the equation of the sphere is given by
$$(x - h)^2 + (y - k)^2 + (z - j)^2 = r^2$$

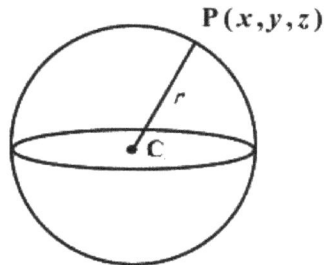

Equation of a Sphere from the Origin

If $P(x,y,z)$ is any point on a sphere with centre at the origin and radius r, then the equation of the sphere is given by $x^2 + y^2 + z^2 = r^2$

General Equation of a Sphere

The equation of a sphere with centre $(-g, -f, -h)$ and radius $\sqrt{g^2 + f^2 + h^2 - c}$ is given by $x^2 + y^2 + z^2 + 2gx + 2fy + 2hz + c = 0$

where g, f, h and c are contants.

Equation of a Sphere Passing Through Two Points

If (x_1, y_1, z_1) and (x_2, y_2, z_2) are the end points of a diameter, then the equation of the sphere is given by

$(x - x_1)(x - x_2) + (y - y_1)(y - y_2) + (z - z_1)(z - z_2) = 0$

Points on a Sphere

In spherical coordinates, the points on the sphere are given by

$x = r \sin\phi\cos\theta$

$y = r \sin\phi\sin\theta$

$z = r\cos\phi$, where $0 \leq \theta \leq 2\pi$, $0 \leq \phi \leq \pi$

Great Circle of a Sphere

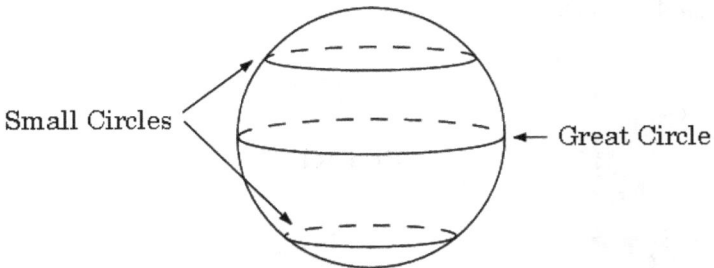

Small Circles ← → Great Circle

The section of a sphere that contains the diameter of the sphere is known as the great circle and the section which does not contain the diameter is known as the small circle.

The great circle divides a sphere into two hemispheres.

Mathematics Formulae

⑦ *Boolean Algebra*

ables are the truth values i.e. true and false which are generally rep-

algebra are conjunction, disjunction and negation.

Statement : A sentence is called a mathematically acceptable statement if it is either true or false but not both.

Statements are generally represented by small letters p, q, r...

Negation of a statement : The denial of a statement is called the negation of the statement.

If p is a statement, then the negation of p is also a statement which is read as 'not p' and is denoted by $\sim p$.

Note : "It is not the case" or "It is false that" are also used while forming the negation of a statement.

Compound Statement : A statement which is made up of two or more statements which are connected by words like 'and', 'or' etc. is called a compound statement.

Connectives : The words like 'and', 'or' etc. which join two statements are called connectives.

(i) The compound statement with 'And' is true if all its component statements are true.

(ii) The component statement with 'And' is false if any of its component statements is false (this includes the case that some of its component statements are false or all of its component statements are false).

Note: A statement with 'And' is not always a compound statement.

(i) A compound statement with an 'Or' is true when one component statement is true or both the component statements are true.

(ii) A compound statement with an 'Or' is false when both the component statements are false.

: The phrases like, 'There exists' and 'For all' are known

Implications

If p then q is the same as the following:

(i) p implies q is denoted by $p \Rightarrow q$. The symbol $\Rightarrow$ stands for implies. For example, a number is a multiple of 9 implies that it is a multiple of 3.

(ii) p is a sufficient condition for q

For example, knowing that a number is a multiple of 9 is sufficient to conclude that it is a multiple of 3

(iii) p only if q

For example, a number is a multiple of 9 only if it is a multiple of 3

(iv) q is a necessary condition for p

For example, when a number is a multiple of 9, it is necessarily a multiple of 3

(v) $\sim q$ implies $\sim p$

For example, if a number is not a multiple of 3, then it is not a multiple of 9

Contrapositive of a Statement

If p then q is the statement if $\sim q$, then $\sim p$

Converse of a Statement

$p \Rightarrow q$ is the statement $q \Rightarrow p$

$p \Rightarrow q$ together with its converse gives p if and only if q.

'*If and only if*', represented by the symbol $\Leftrightarrow$ means the following equivalent forms for the given statements p and q.

(i) p if and only if q

(ii) q if and only if p

(iii) p is necessary and sufficient condition for q and vice-versa

(iv) $p \Leftrightarrow q$

Validity of Statements

The following methods are used to check the validity of statements:

(i) direct method

(ii) contrapositive method

(iii) method of contradiction

(iv) using a counter example

Direct Method

Rule 1 : Statements with 'And'

If p and q are mathematical statements, then in order to show that the statement 'p and q' is true, the following steps are followed.

Step-1 : Show that the statement p is true.

Step-2 : Show that the statement q is true.

Rule 2 : Statements with 'Or'

If p and q are mathematical statements, then in order to show that the statement 'p or q' is true, one must consider the following.

Case 1 : By assuming that p is false, show that q must be true.

Case 2 : By assuming that q is false, show that p must be true.

Rule 3 : Statements with 'If-then'

In order to prove the statement 'if p then q' we need to show that any one of the following cases is true.

Case 1 : By assuming that p is true, prove that q must be true.
(Direct method)

Case 2 : By assuming that q is false, prove that p must be false.

Contrapositive Method

Rule 4 : Statements with 'if and only if'

In order to prove the statement 'p if and only if q', we need to show.

(i) If p is true, then q is true

and

(ii) If q is true, then p is true.

Contradiction Method

To check whether a statement p is true, we assume that p is not true i.e. $\sim p$ is true. Then, we arrive at some result which contradicts our assumption. Therefore, we conclude that p is true.

Counter Example

In mathematics, counter examples are used to disprove the statement. However, generating example in favour of a statement does not provide validity of the statement.

Truth Table

A truth table shows how a logic circuit's output responds to various combinations of the inputs using logic 1 for true and logic 0 for false.

Notation

The following notation is used for Boolean algebra :

False: 0

True: 1

Basic Operations

– Conjunction / xAND y : $x \cdot y / x \wedge y$

– Disjunction / x OR y : $x + y / x \vee y$

– Negation / Complement / NOT : $\sim x / \bar{x}$

x OR y: $x \oplus y$ (Exclusive OR is represented by XOR)

Exclusive disjunction or *exclusive OR* is a logical operation that outputs true whenever both inputs differ (one is true, the other is false).

Logical Identity

P	p
Operand	Value
T	T
F	F

Logical Negation

P	$\sim p$
T	F
F	T

Logical Conjunction

P	q	$p \wedge q$
T	T	T
T	F	F
F	T	F
F	F	F

Logical Disjunction

P	q	$p \vee q$
T	T	T
T	F	T
F	T	T
F	F	F

Exclusive Disjunction

p	q	$p \oplus q$
T	T	F
T	F	T
F	T	T
F	F	F

Logical Implication

p	q	$p \Rightarrow q$
T	T	T
T	F	F
F	T	T
F	F	T

Logical Equality

p	q	$p \equiv q$
T	T	T
T	F	F
F	T	F
F	F	T

De Morgan's Laws

(i) The negation of a conjunction is the disjunction of the negations.
   i.e. 'not (A and B)' is the same as '(not A) or (not B)'

(ii) The negation of a disjunction is the conjunction of the negations.
   'not (A or B)' is the same as '(not A) and (not B)'

Basic laws of Boolean Algebra

Constant

NOT	AND	OR	XOR
$\bar{0} = 1$	$0 \cdot 0 = 0$	$0 + 0 = 0$	$0 \oplus 0 = 0$
$\bar{1} = 0$	$0 \cdot 1 = 0$	$0 + 1 = 1$	$0 \oplus 1 = 1$

	$1 \cdot 0 = 0$	$1 + 0 = 1$	$1 \oplus 0 = 1$
	$1 \cdot 1 = 1$	$1 + 1 = 1$	$1 \oplus 1 = 0$

Constant and Variable

AND	OR	XOR	
$0 \cdot x = 0$	$0 + x = x$	$0 \oplus x = x$	
$1 \cdot x = x$	$1 + x = 1$	$1 \oplus x = \bar{x}$	

One variable

NOT	AND	OR	XOR
$\text{NOT}\,\bar{x} = x$	$x \cdot x = x$	$x + x = x$	$x \oplus x = x$
	$x \cdot \bar{x} = 0$	$x + \bar{x} = 1$	$x \oplus \bar{x} = 1$

XOR

XOR can be defined in terms of AND, OR, NOT:

$$x \oplus y = (x \cdot \bar{y}) + (\bar{x} \cdot y)$$
$$x \oplus y = (x + y) \cdot (\bar{x} + \bar{y})$$
$$x \oplus y = (x + y) \cdot \overline{(x.y)}$$

Commutativity	Associativity	Distributivity
AND: $x \cdot y = y \cdot x$	AND: $(x \cdot y) \cdot z$ $= x \cdot (y \cdot z)$	$x \cdot (y+z) = (x \cdot y) + (x \cdot z)$
OR: $x + y = y + x$	OR: $(x + y) + z$ $= x + (y + z)$	$x + (y \cdot z)$ $= (x + y) \cdot (x + z)$
XOR: $x \oplus y = y \oplus x$	XOR: $(x \oplus y) \oplus z$ $= x \oplus (y \oplus z)$	$x \cdot (y \oplus z)$ $= (x \cdot y) \oplus (x \cdot z)$

De Morgan's laws

NAND: $\overline{x \cdot y} = \bar{x} + \bar{y}$
NOR: $\overline{x + y} = \bar{x} \cdot \bar{y}$

Mathematics Formulae

8

Vectors Formulae

SCALAR AND VECTOR

A quantity that has only magnitude is known as a scalar quantity.

A quantity that has magnitude as well as direction is known as a vector quantity. A vector PQ is represented as $\overline{PQ}$ (vector PQ) or a (vector a). The arrowhead indicates the direction of the vector.

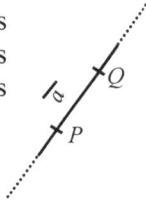

point.

known as the _____ or *magnitude* of a vector. It is represented by $\overline{PQ}$ or $|a|$.

The position vector of a point P with coordinates (
by

$$r = \left|\overline{OP}\right| = \sqrt{x^2 + y^2 + z^2}$$

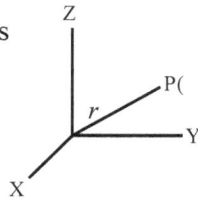

_____ : A vector whose initial and terminal points coincide is known as a null vector or zero vector. It is represented by ___ . A null vector can have any direction.

Unit Vector : A vector whose magnitude is unity is called a unit vector. The unit vector having the same direction as that of a given vector a (a) is represented by $\hat{a}$ (a cap).

_____ : Two vectors a and ___ are said to be equal, if they have the same magnitude and the same direction.

_____ : Two or more vectors having the same initial point are called co-initial vectors.

Co-planar and Non-coplanar Vectors : Three or more vectors are said to be co-planar when they are parallel to the same plane. Otherwise they are said to be non-coplanar vectors.

Collinear Vectors and Non-collinear Vectors : Two or more vectors are said to be collinear if they are parallel to the same straight line, irrespective of their magnitudes and directions. Otherwise they are said to be non-collinear vectors.

Like and Unlike Vectors : Collinear vectors having the same direction are called like vectors. Collinear vectors having the opposite direction are called unlike vectors.

Negative of a Vector : A vector whose magnitude is the same as that of a given vector and the direction is opposite to that of it is known as negative of a vector. $\overline{QP}$ (vector QP) is the negative of $\overline{PQ}$ (vector PQ).

Inclination of Vectors

The angle θ between two vectors $\vec{a}$ and $\vec{b}$ is known as the inclination of vectors ($0 \le \theta \le \pi$).

If $\theta = \pi/2$, the vectors are said to be *orthogonal* or perpendicular.

If $\theta = 0$ or π, the vectors are said to be parallel or coincident.

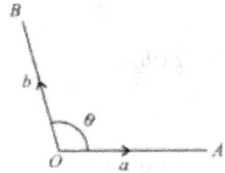

Addition of Vectors

Triangle Law of Vector Addition

Triangle law of vector states that if two vectors can be represented both in magnitude and direction by two sides of a triangle taken in the same order, then their resultant is represented both in magnitude and direction by the third side of the triangle taken in the reverse order (opposite direction).

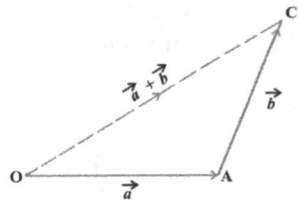

$$\overline{OC} = \overline{OA} + \overline{AC} \text{ or } \overline{OC} = \vec{a} + \vec{b}$$

Note: The vector sum of three sides of a triangle taken in order is zero vector.

Parallelogram Law of Vector Addition

Parallelogram law of vector states that if two vectors can be represented both in magnitude and direction by two adjacent sides of a parallelogram drawn from the

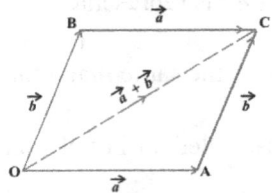

same point (co-initial vectors), then their resultant is represented both in magnitude and direction by the diagonal passing through the same point.

If $\overline{OA}$ and $\overline{OB}$ represent two vectors $\vec{a}$ and $\vec{b}$ respectively drawn from the point O, then the resultant is given by the diagonal $OC(\vec{a}+\vec{b})$.

Properties of Vector Addition

(i) *Commutative Property*
   For any two vectors $\vec{a}$ and $\vec{b}$, $+ \vec{b} = \vec{b} + \vec{a}$

(ii) *Associative Property*
   For any three vectors $\vec{a}$, $\vec{b}$ and $\vec{c}$,
   $$(\vec{a}+\vec{b})+\vec{c} = \vec{a}+(\vec{b}+\vec{c})$$

(iii)*Additive Identity*
   Zero vector is the additive identity.
   For every vector $\vec{a}$, $\vec{a} + 0 = 0 + \vec{a} = \vec{a}$

(iv)*Additive Inverse*
   For any vector $\vec{a}$ there exists a vector $-\vec{a}$ such that
   $$\vec{a} + (-\vec{a}) = (-\vec{a}) + \vec{a} = 0$$

Multiplication of a Vector by a Scalar

If $\vec{a}$ is any vector and λ is a scalar, then the product $\lambda\vec{a}$ is known as the multiplication of a vector by a scalar.

(i) $\lambda\vec{a}$ is a vector which is collinear to $\vec{a}$.

(ii) If λ is positive, vector $\lambda\vec{a}$ has the same direction as $\vec{a}$.

(iii)If λ is negative, vector $\lambda\vec{a}$ has the direction opposite to $\vec{a}$.

(iv)$|\lambda\vec{a}| = |\lambda||\vec{a}|$

(v) For any scalar λ, $\lambda\vec{0} = 0$.

(vi) For a given vector $\vec{a}$, the unit vector in the direction of $\vec{a}$ is given by
   $$\hat{a} = \frac{1}{|\vec{a}|}\vec{a}, \text{ where } \vec{a} \neq 0$$

Components of a Vector

Let $\hat{i}$, $\hat{j}$, $\hat{k}$ be the position vectors along x, y and z axis respectively. The position vector of a point R(x, y, z) with respect to the origin known as component form of a vector is given by

$$\vec{r} = x\hat{i} + y\hat{j} + z\hat{k}$$

x, y and z are known as the *scalar components* or rectangular components of $\vec{r}$.

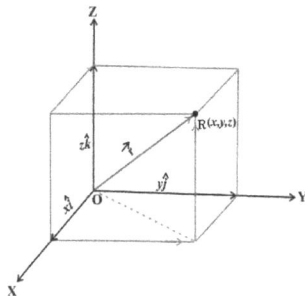

$x\hat{i}$, $y\hat{j}$ and $z\hat{k}$ are known as the *vector components* of $\vec{r}$.

Length of Component Vector

The length of component vector $\vec{r} = x\hat{i} + y\hat{j} + z\hat{k}$ is given by

$$|\vec{r}| = |x\hat{i} + y\hat{j} + z\hat{k}| = \sqrt{x^2 + y^2 + z^2}$$

Properties of Component Vector

If $\vec{a} = a_1\hat{i} + a_2\hat{j} + a_3\hat{k}$ and $\vec{b} = b_1\hat{i} + b_2\hat{j} + b_3\hat{k}$ be two component vectors, then

(i) the two vectors and $\vec{b}$ are equal if and only if

$a_1 = b_1$, $a_2 = b_2$, $a_3 = b_3$

(ii) the sum of the vectors is given by

$$\vec{a} + \vec{b} = (a_1 + b_1)\hat{i} + (a_2 + b_2)\hat{j} + (a_3 + b_3)\hat{k}$$

(iii) The difference of the vectors is given by

$$\vec{a} - \vec{b} = (a_1 - b_1)\hat{i} + (a_2 - b_2)\hat{j} + (a_3 - b_3)\hat{k}$$

(iv) The product of any vector $\vec{a}$ by a scalar λ is given by

$$\lambda\vec{a} = (\lambda a_1)\hat{i} + (\lambda a_2)\hat{j} + (\lambda a_3)\hat{k}$$

(v) The dot product of two vectors $\vec{a}$ and $\vec{b}$ is given by

$$\vec{a} \cdot \vec{b} = a_1 b_1 + a_2 b_2 + a_3 b_3$$

Distributive Laws

If $\vec{a}$ and $\vec{b}$ are two vectors, m and n are two scalars, then

(i) $m(\vec{a} + \vec{b}) = m\vec{a} + m\vec{b}$

(ii) $m(n\vec{a}) = (mn)\vec{a}$

(iii) $m\vec{a} + n\vec{a} = (m + n)\vec{a}$

Direction Ratio and Direction Cosine

If $\vec{a} = a_1\hat{i} + a_2\hat{j} + a_3\hat{k}$, then a_1, a_2 and a_3 are called direction ratios.

If l, m, n are direction cosines of a vector, then

$l\hat{i} + m\hat{j} + n\hat{k} = (\cos\alpha)\hat{i} + (\cos\beta)\hat{j} + (\cos\gamma)\hat{k}$ is the unit vector in the direction of that vector, where α, β and γ are the angles which the vector makes with x, y and z axes respectively.

Vector Joining Two Points

If $P(x_1, y_1, z_1)$ and $Q(x_2, y_2, z_2)$ are any two points, then the vector joining the points P and Q is given by

$$\overline{PQ} = \sqrt{(x_2 - x_1)^2 + (y_2 - y_1)^2 + (z_2 - z_1)^2}$$

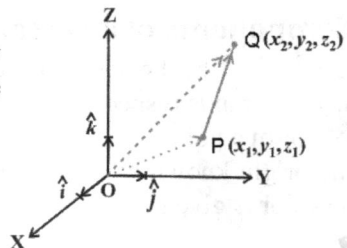

Section Formula

Internal Division

The position vector ($\vec{r}$) of a point R dividing a line segment joining points A and B whose position vectors with respect to the origin are $\vec{a}$ and $\vec{b}$ respectively, internally in the ratio $m : n$ is given by

$$\vec{r} = \frac{m\vec{b} + n\vec{a}}{m + n}$$

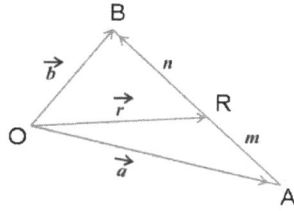

External Division

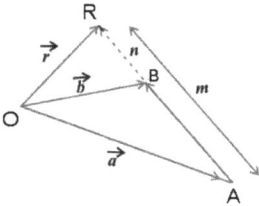

The position vector ($\vec{r}$) of a point R dividing a line segment joining points A and B whose position vectors with respect to the origin are $\vec{a}$ and $\vec{b}$ respectively, externally in the ratio $m : n$ is given by

$$\vec{r} = \frac{m\vec{b} - n\vec{a}}{m - n}$$

Mid Point Formula

If R is the mid point of AB, then $m = n$. Hence, by internal division formula we get,

$$\vec{r} = \frac{\vec{a} + \vec{b}}{2}$$

Scalar (or dot) Product of Two Vectors

The scalar product of two non zero vectors $\vec{a}$ and $\vec{b}$ represented by $a \cdot b$ is given by $\vec{a} \cdot \vec{b} = |\vec{a}||\vec{b}| \cos\theta$ where θ is the angle between two vectors $\vec{a}$ and $\vec{b}$, $(0 \leq \theta \leq \pi)$.

(i) If $\theta = 0$, $\vec{a} \cdot \vec{b} = |\vec{a}||\vec{b}|$

(ii) If $\theta = \pi$, $\vec{a} \cdot \vec{b} = -|\vec{a}||\vec{b}|$

Properties of Scalar Product (Two Vectors)

(i) $\vec{a} \cdot \vec{b}$ is a real number.

(ii) $\vec{a} \cdot \vec{b} = 0$ if and only if $\vec{a}$ and $\vec{b}$ are perpendicular to each other.

(iii) Commutative Property

If $\vec{a}$ and $\vec{b}$ are two non zero vectors, then $\vec{a} \cdot \vec{b} = \vec{b} \cdot \vec{a}$

(iv) Distributive Property

For any three vectors $\vec{a}$, $\vec{b}$ and $\vec{c}$, $\vec{a} \cdot (\vec{b} + \vec{c}) = \vec{a} \cdot \vec{b} + \vec{a} \cdot \vec{c}$

(v) The angle between two non zero vectors $\vec{a}$ and $\vec{b}$ is given by

$$\cos\theta = \frac{\vec{a} \cdot \vec{b}}{|\vec{a}||\vec{b}|}, \text{ or } \theta = \cos^{-1}\left(\frac{\vec{a} \cdot \vec{b}}{|\vec{a}||\vec{b}|}\right)$$

(vi) If $\vec{a}$ and $\vec{b}$ are any two vectors and λ is a scalar, then

$$(\lambda\vec{a}) \cdot \vec{b} = (\lambda\vec{a}) \cdot \vec{b} = \lambda(\vec{a} \cdot \vec{b}) = \vec{a} \cdot (\lambda\vec{b})$$

(vii) *Property of Unit Vector*

If $\hat{i}, \hat{j}, \hat{k}$ are mutually perpendicular unit vectors, then

$$\hat{i} \cdot \hat{i} = \hat{j} \cdot \hat{j} = \hat{k} \cdot \hat{k} = 1$$
$$\hat{i} \cdot \hat{j} = \hat{j} \cdot \hat{k} = \hat{k} \cdot \hat{i} = 0$$

Projection of a Vector on a Line

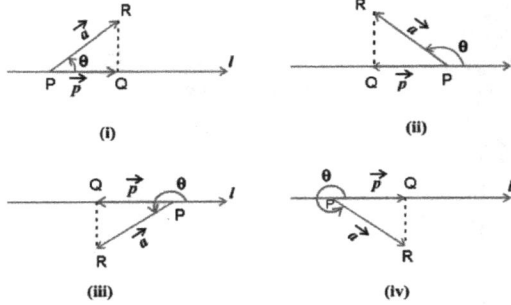

(i)

(ii)

(iii)

(iv)

(i) $0 < \theta < \pi/2$
(ii) $\pi/2 < \theta < \pi$
(iii) $\pi < \theta < 3\pi/2$
(iv) $3\pi/2 < \theta < 2\pi$

- Let vector PR make an angle θ with a directed line l, in the anti-clockwise direction. Then the projection vector of PR $(\vec{p})$ on l is given by $\vec{p} = |\overrightarrow{PR}| \cos\theta$

- If $\cos\theta$ is positive, the direction of $(\vec{p})$ is same as that of line l.

- If $\cos\theta$ is negative, the direction of $(\vec{p})$ is opposite to that of line l.

Properties of Projection of a Vector on a Line

(i) If $\theta = 0$, the projection vector of $\overline{PQ}$ is $\overline{PQ}$ itself.

(ii) If $\theta = \dfrac{\pi}{2}$, the projection vector of $\overline{PQ}$ is zero vector.

(iii) If $\theta = \pi$, the projection vector of $\overline{PQ}$ is $\overline{QP}$

(iv) If $\theta = \dfrac{3\pi}{2}$, the projection vector of $\overline{PQ}$ is zero vector.

(v) Projection of a vector say $\vec{a}$ on another vector say $\vec{b}$, is given by

$$\vec{a} \cdot \hat{b} \text{ or } \vec{a} \cdot \left(\dfrac{\vec{b}}{|\vec{b}|} \right) \text{ or } \dfrac{1}{|\vec{b}|} (\vec{a} \cdot \vec{b})$$

Cauchy Schwartz Inequality

For any two vectors $\vec{a}$ and $\vec{b}$, $|\vec{a}.\vec{b}| \leq |\vec{a}||\vec{b}|$

Triangle Inequality

For any two vectors $\vec{a}$ and $\vec{b}$, $|\vec{a}+\vec{b}| \leq |\vec{a}| + |\vec{b}|$

Vector (or cross) Product of Two Vectors

The vector product of two non zero vectors $\vec{a}$ and $\vec{b}$ represented by $\vec{a} \times \vec{b}$ is given by $\vec{a} \times \vec{b} = |\vec{a}||\vec{b}| \sin\theta \, \hat{n}$ where θ is the angle between two vectors $\vec{a}$ and $\vec{b}$, $(0 \leq \theta \leq \pi)$ and $\hat{n}$ is a unit vector perpendicular to both $\vec{a}$ and $\vec{b}$, such that $\vec{a}$, $\vec{b}$ and $\hat{n}$ form a right handed system.

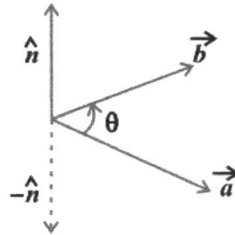

(i) If $\theta = 0$, $\vec{a} \times \vec{b} = 0$

(ii) If $\theta = \dfrac{\pi}{2}$, $\vec{a} \times \vec{b} = |\vec{a}||\vec{b}|$

Properties of Vector Product (Two vectors)

(i) $\vec{a} \times \vec{b}$ is a vector.

(ii) $\vec{a} \times \vec{b} = 0$ if and only if $\vec{a}$ and $\vec{b}$ are parallel to each other.

(iii) *Commutative Property*

Vector Product is not commutative. If $\vec{a}$ and $\vec{b}$ are two vectors then $\vec{a} \times \vec{b} \neq \vec{b} \times \vec{a}$, $\vec{a} \times \vec{b} = -\vec{b} \times \vec{a}$.

(iv) *Distributive Property*

For any three vectors , $\vec{b}$, $\vec{c}$ and a scalar λ,

$\vec{a} \times (\vec{b} + \vec{c}) = \vec{a} \times \vec{b} + \vec{a} \times \vec{c}$

(v) If $\vec{a}$ and $\vec{b}$ are any two vectors and λ is a scalar then

$\lambda(\vec{a} \times \vec{b}) = (\lambda\vec{a}) \times \vec{b} = \vec{a} \times (\lambda\vec{b})$

(vi) The angle between two vectors $\vec{a}$ and $\vec{b}$ is given by

$\sin\theta = \dfrac{|\vec{a} \times \vec{b}|}{|\vec{a}||\vec{b}|}$ or $\theta = \sin^{-1}\left(\dfrac{|\vec{a} \times \vec{b}|}{|\vec{a}||\vec{b}|}\right)$

(vii) *Property of Unit Vector*

If $\hat{i}, \hat{j}, \hat{k}$ are mutually perpendicular unit vectors, then

$\hat{i} \times \hat{i} = \hat{j} \times \hat{j} = \hat{k} \times \hat{k} = \hat{0}$

$\hat{i} \times \hat{j} = \hat{k}, \ \hat{j} \times \hat{k} = \hat{i}, \ \hat{k} \times \hat{i} = \hat{j}$

Vector Product of Component Vectors

If $\vec{a} = a_1\hat{i} + a_2\hat{j} + a_3\hat{k}$ and $\vec{b} = b_1\hat{i} + b_2\hat{j} + b_3\hat{k}$ be two component vectors, then their cross product is given by

$$\vec{a} \times \vec{b} = \begin{vmatrix} \hat{i} & \hat{j} & \hat{k} \\ a_1 & a_2 & a_3 \\ b_1 & b_2 & b_3 \end{vmatrix}$$

Area of a Triangle

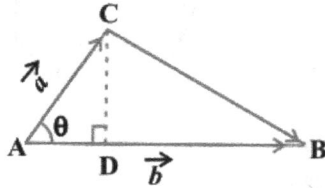

If $\vec{a}$ and $\vec{b}$ are two adjacent sides of a triangle, then

Area of tringle $= \dfrac{1}{2}|\vec{a} \times \vec{b}|$

Area of a Parallelogram

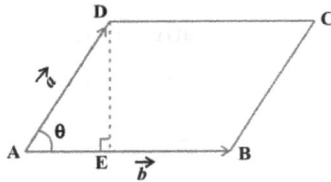

If $\vec{a}$ and $\vec{b}$ are two adjacent sides of a parallelogram, then

Area of parallelogram $= |\vec{a} \times \vec{b}|$

Mathematics Formulae

Statistics Formulae

PERMUTATION AND COMBINATION

If an event can occur in *m* different ways, following which another event can occur in *n* different ways, then the total number of occurrence of the events in the given order is   .

For three events

If an event can occur in *m* different ways, following which another event can occur in *n* different ways, following which a third event can occur in *p* different ways, then the total number of occurrence of the events in the given order is   .

Note:

number of events.

n

n' natural numbers is called factorial *n* and is deonoted by *n*! i.e,

n		*n* −	*n*
n! =	!		
n! =		! if *n*	
n! =			! if *n*

Note:

-

jects taken some or all at a time.

Linear Permutation

A permutation is said to be a linear permutation if the objects are arranged in a line. A linear permutation is simply called as a permutation.

Circular Permutation

A permutation is said to be a circular permutation if the objects are arranged in the form of a circle.

Formula for Linear Permutation

The number of (linear) permutations that can be formed by taking r things at a time from a set of n distinct things ($r \leq n$) is denoted by ^nP_r or $P(n, r)$.

$^nP_r = n(n-1)(n-2)(n-3)......(n-r+1)$

where $0 < r \leq n$

$^nP_r = \dfrac{n!}{(n-r)!}, \; 0 \leq r \leq n$

Note:

$^nP_n = n!$ and $^nP_0 = 1$

Number of Permutations Under Certain Conditions

(i) The number of permutations of n objects, where p objects are of the same kind and rest are all different $= \dfrac{n!}{p!}$

(ii) The number of permutations of n objects, where p_1 objects are of one kind, p_2 are of second kind, ..., p_k are of kth kind and the rest, if any, are of different kind is $\dfrac{n!}{p_1! p_2! ... p_k!}$

(iii) Number of permutations of n dissimilar things, taken r at a time, when a particular thing is to be always included in each arrangement, is $r\left(^{n-1}P_{r-1}\right)$

(iv) Number of permutations of n different things, taken r at a time, when a particular thing is never taken in each arrangement is $^{n-1}P_r$

(v) Number of permutations of n different things, taken all at a time, when m specified things always come together is $m!(n-m+1)!$.

(vi) Number of permutations of n different things, taken all at a time, when m specified never come together is $n! - [m!(n-m+1)!]$.

(vii) The number of permutations of n dissimilar things taken r at a time when $k(<r)$ particular things always occur is $[^{n-k}P_{r-k}] \cdot [^rP_k]$.

(viii) The number of permutations of n dissimilar things taken r at a time when k particular things never occur is $^{n-k}P_r$

(ix) The number of permutations of n different objects taken r at a time when repetition is allowed any number of times is n^r

(x) The number of permutations of n different things, taken not more than r at a time, when each thing may occur any number of times is

$$n + n^2 + n^3 + \ldots\ldots + n^r = \frac{n(n^r - 1)}{n - 1}$$

(xi) The number of permutations of n different things taken not more than r at a time ${}^nP_1 + {}^nP_2 + {}^nP_3 + \ldots + {}^nP_r$

Circular Permutation

(i) The number of circular permutations of n dissimilar things taken r at a time when clockwise and anticlockwise orders are taken as different is $\frac{{}^nP_r}{r}$.

(ii) The number of circular permutations of n dissimilar things taken all at a time is $(n - 1)!$

(iii) The number of circular permutations of n things taken r at a time in one direction is $\frac{{}^nP_r}{2r}$.

(iv) The number of circular permutations of n dissimilar things in clock-wise direction = Number of permutations in anticlock-wise direction = $\frac{(n-1)!}{2}$.

Combination

A selection that can be formed by taking some or all of a finite set of objects is known as combination.

The number of combinations of n dissimilar things taken r at a time is denoted by ${}^nC_r$ or $C(n, r)$ or $\binom{n}{r}$.

Relationship Between Permutation and Combination

${}^nP_r = {}^nC_r \, r!$ where $0 < r \le n$

Relationship of Combination

(i) ${}^nC_r = \dfrac{n!}{r!(n-r)!}$, $0 < r \le n$

(ii) ${}^nC_r = {}^nC_{r-1}$

(iii) ${}^nC_{n-r} = {}^nC_r$

(iv) ${}^nC_r + {}^nC_{r-1} = {}^{n+1}C_r$

(v) *If* ${}^nC_r = {}^nC_s \Rightarrow r = s$ or $n = r + s$

(vi) The number of combinations of n things taken r at a time in which
   a) s particular things will always occur is ${}^{n-s}C_{r-s}$
   b) s particular things will never occur is ${}^{n-s}C_r$

c) s particular things always occur and p particular things never occur is $^{n-p-s}C_{r-s}$

(vii) $^nC + {}^nC_1 + {}^nC_2 + ... + {}^nC_n = 2^n$

(viii) $^nC + {}^nC_2 + {}^nC_4 + ... = {}^nC_1 + {}^nC_3 + {}^nC_5 + ... = 2^{n-1}$

Note:

$$^nC_n = {}^nC = 1 \text{ and } {}^nC_1 = n$$

(i) Number of ways in which $(m + n)$ items can be divided into two unequal groups containing m and n items is $^{m+n}C_m = \dfrac{(m+n)!}{m!n!}$.

(ii) The number of ways in which mn different items can be divided equally into m groups, each containing n objects and the order of the groups is not important is $\left[\dfrac{(mn)!}{(n!)^m} \right] \dfrac{1}{m!}$

(iii) The number of ways in which mn different items can be divided equally into m groups, each containing n objects and the order of the groups is important is $\dfrac{(mn)!}{(n!)^m}$.

(iv) The number of ways in which $(m + n + p)$ things can be divided into three different groups of   and p things respectively is $\dfrac{(m+n+p)!}{m!n!p!}$.

PROBABILITY

In Mathematics, Probability is the calculation of uncertainty. It is the measure of how likely an event occurs.

Experiment : An action that has various outcomes that occur unpre-

For example, throw of a dice.

          : An outcome is the possible result of a single trial of an experiment. For example, tossing of a coin has two possible outcomes – heads or tails.

          : The collection of all possible outcomes of a random experiment is known as sample space. For example, sample space in

point.

Event : An event is one or more outcomes of an experiment. For ex-

Mathematics Formulae

ample, getting an even number in the throw of a dice. An event is a subset of the sample space.

Experimental or Empirical Probability : Probabilities based on the results of actual experiments and adequate recordings of the happening of the events are known as experimental or empirical probability.

Theoretical Probability or *Classical Probability* : The probability that a certain outcome will occur as determined through reasoning or calculation is known as theoretical probability.

Probability of an Event

If the experiments have an equally likely outcome, then the classical probability or theoretical probability of an event is given by

$$\text{Probability of an event} = \frac{\text{Number of favourable outcomes}}{\text{Total number of outcomes}}$$

Important Points on Cards

♦ A deck of playing cards consists of 52 cards which are divided into 4 suits - spades (♠), hearts (♥), diamonds (♦) and clubs (♣).

♦ Two suits are black (clubs and spades) while two are red (hearts and diamonds) in colour.

♦ Each suit consists of 13 cards namely ace, 2, 3, 4, 5, 6, 7, 8, 9, 10, Jack, Queen and King.

♦ Kings, queens and jacks are called face cards.

Types of Event

Impossible Event : An empty set is an impossible event.

Sure Event : The whole sample space is a sure event.

Simple Event or Elementary Event : An event having only one outcome is called an elementary event.

Compound Event : If an event has more than one sample point, it is known as a compound event.

Algebra of Events

Complimentary Event : For every event A there corresponds not an event A which is known as complement of A. The complement of A is represented by A' or A^c. If S is the sample space, then

A' = S – A = {a : a ∈ S and a ∉ A}

The Event 'A and B' : If A and B are two events, then the set A ∩ B denotes the event 'A and B'.

A ∩ B = {a : a ∈ A and a ∈ B}

The Event 'A or B' : If A and B are two events, then the set A ∪ B denotes the event 'A or B'.

$A \cup B = \{a : a \in A \text{ or } a \in B\}$

The Event 'A but not B' : If A and B are two events, then the set $A \cap B'$ denotes the event 'A but not B'. It is represented by $A - B$.

$A - B = A \cap B'$

Mutually Exclusive Events

If A and B are two events, then they are called mutually exclusive if they cannot occur simultaneously i.e. if the occurrence of any one of them excludes the occurrence of the other event.

$$A \cap B = \phi, \text{ (A and B are disjoint sets)}$$

Exhaustive Events

(i) Let S be the sample space and E_1, E_2, ..., E_n be n events. If
$E_1 \cup E_2 \cup E_3 \cup ... \cup E_n = \overset{n}{\underset{i=1}{\cup}} E_i = S$, then E_1, E_2, ..., E_n are called exhaustive events.

(ii) If $E_i \cap E_j = \phi$ for $i \neq j$ and $\overset{n}{\underset{i=1}{\cup}} E_i = S$, then events E_1, E_2, ..., E_n are called mutually exclusive and exhaustive events.

Some Results of Probability

(i) The sum of the probabilities of all possible outcomes of an event of an experiment is 1.

(ii) P(event) + P(not event) = 1

(iii) Probability of an event always lies between 0 and 1 or $0 \leq P(\text{event}) \leq 1$

(vi) Probability of an impossible event is 0, $P(\phi) = 0$

(v) Probability of a sure event is 1.

(vi) If S be the sample space containing elements a_1, a_2,..., a_n, then

(i) $P(a_1) + P(a_2) + ... + P(a_n) = 1$

(ii) $0 \leq P(a_i) \leq 1$ for each $a_i \in S$

(iii) For any event A, $P(A) = \sum P(a_i)$, $a_i \in A$

Probability Rules

(i) If A and B are any two events of a sample space associated with a random experiment, then the probability the event A or event B occurs is given by: $P(A \cup B) = P(A) + P(B) - P(A \cap B)$

(ii) If two events A and B of a random experiment are mutually exclusive, then
$$P(A \cup B) = P(A) + P(B) \text{ and } P(A \cap B) = 0$$

(iii) If A and B – A are mutually exclusive, then
$$P(A \cup B) = P(A) + P(B - A)$$

(iv) If A ∩ B and B – A are mutually exclusive
$$P(B) = P(A \cap B) + P(B - A)$$
(v) $P(A^C) + P(A) = 1$
or $P(\text{not A}) = P(A^c) = P(A') = 1 - P(A)$
where $P(A^C)$ and P(A') denote the probability of A complement.
(vi) If A, B, C are three events of a sample space associated with a random experiment, then
$$P(A \cup B \cup C) = P(A) + P(B) + P(C) - P(A \cap B) - P(A \cap C)$$
$$- P(B \cap C) + P(A \cap B \cap C)$$

Conditional Probability

If A and B are two events of a sample space associated with a random experiment, the conditional probability of the event A given that B has occurred is denoted by P(A | B). It is given by

$$P(A | B) = \frac{P(A \cap B)}{P(B)} \text{ where } P(B) \neq 0$$

Properties of Conditional Probability

(i) If A and B are two events of a sample space S associated with a random experiment, then P(S | B) = P(B | B) = 1
(ii) If A and B are any two events of a sample space S associated with a random experiment and C is an event of S such that P(C) ≠ 0, then
$$P((A \cup B) | C) = P(A | C) + P(B | C) - P((A \cap B) | C)$$
(iii) If A and B are disjoint events, then
$$P((A \cup B) | C) = P(A | C) + P(B | C) \text{ and } P((A \cap B) | C) = 0$$
(iv) If A and B are two events of a sample space S associated with a random experiment and B ≠ φ, then
$$P(A' | B) = 1 - P(A|B)$$

Multiplication Theorem of Probability

(i) If A and B are any two events of a sample space associated with a random experiment, then the probability that the event A and event B both occur is given by:
(a) $P(A \cap B) = P(A) P(B|A)$ where $P(A) \neq 0$
(b) $P(A \cap B) = P(B) P(A|B)$ where $P(B) \neq 0$
(ii) If A, B and C are any three events of a sample space associated with a random experiment, then the probability that the event A, event B and event C all occur is given by:
(a) $P(A \cap B \cap C) = P(A) P(B|A) P(C | (A \cap B))$
(b) $P(A \cap B \cap C) = P(A) P(B|A) P(C | (AB))$

Independent Events

(i) Two events A and B of a sample space associated with a random experiment are known as independent events if the probability of occurrence of one of them is not affected by the occurrence of the other.

(ii) Two events A and B of a sample space associated with a random experiment are independent if $P(A \mid B) = P(A)$ where $P(B) \neq 0$ and $P(B \mid A) = P(B)$ where $P(A) \neq 0$

(iii) Two events A and B of a sample space associated with a random experiment are independent if
$$P(A \cap B) = P(A)P(B)$$

(iv) Three events A, B and C of a sample space associated with a random experiment are said to be mutually independent, if
$$P(A \cap B) = P(A)P(B)$$
$$P(A \cap C) = P(A)P(C)$$
$$P(B \cap C) = P(B)P(C)$$
and $P(A \cap B \cap C) = P(A)P(B)P(C)$

Note:

Two events A and B of a sample space associated with a random experiment are said to be dependent if $P(A \cap B) \neq P(A)P(B)$

Properties of Independent Event

If two events A and B of a sample space associated with a random experiment are independent then,

(i) A and B' are independent

(ii) A' and B are independent

(iii) A' and B' are independent

(iv) P(at least one of A and B) $= 1 - P(A') P(B')$

Partition of a Sample Space

The events $E_1, E_2, ..., E_n$ represent a partition of the sample space S if they are pairwise disjoint, exhaustive and have nonzero probabilities.

Theorem of Total Probability

Let A be any event associated with sample space S and let $\{ E_1, E_2, ..., E_n \}$ be a partition of the sample space such that each of the events $E_1, E_2, ..., E_n$ has non zero probabilities then
$$P(A) = P(E_1) P(A|E_1) + P(E_2) P(A|E_2) + ... + P(E_n) P(A|E_n)$$
$$= \sum_{j=1}^{n} P(E_j)P(A \mid E_j)$$

Mathematics Formulae

Bayes' Theorem

If A is any event of non zero probability, E_1, E_2, ..., E_n are n non empty events which constitute a partition of sample space S, i.e. E_1, E_2, ..., E_n are pairwise disjoint and

$$E_1 \cup E_2 \cup E_3 \cup \ldots \cup E_n = \overset{n}{\underset{i=1}{\cup}} E_i = S, \text{ then}$$

$$P(E_i|A) = \frac{P(E_i)\, P(A|E_i)}{\sum\limits_{j=1}^{n} P(E_j)\, P(A|E_j)} \quad \text{for any } i = 1, 2, 3, \ldots, n$$

The events E_1, E_2, ..., E_n are called *hypotheses*.

The probability $P(E_i)$ is called the *priori probability* of the hypothesis E_i

The conditional probability $P(E_i|A)$ is called a *posteriori probability* of the hypothesis E_i.

Random Variable

A random variable is a real valued function whose domain is the sample space of a random experiment.

Probability Distribution of a Random Variable

The probability distribution of a random variable X is the system of numbers

$$X : x_1 \quad x_2 \quad \ldots \quad x_n$$
$$P(X) : p_1 \quad p_2 \quad \ldots \quad p_n$$

where $p_i > 0$, $\sum\limits_{i=1}^{n} p_i = 1$, $i = 1, 2, \ldots, n$

The real numbers x_1, x_2, ..., x_n are the possible values of the random variable X and $p_i (i = 1, 2, \ldots, n)$ is the probability of the random variable X taking the value x_i i.e., $P(X = x_i) = p_i$

Mean of a Random Variable

Let X be a random variable with possible values x_1, x_2, ..., x_n occurring with probabilities p_1, p_2, ..., p_n respectively. The mean of X is denoted by μ. The mean of a random variable X is also called the expectation of X. It is represented by $E(X)$ and given by the equation.

$$E(X) = \mu = \sum\limits_{i=1}^{n} x_i p_i = x_1 p_1 + x_2 p_2 + \ldots + x_n p_n$$

Let X be a random variable with possible values x_1 x_2 x_n occurring with probabilities $_1$ $_2$ $_n$ the mean of the random variable, then the variance is given by

$$\sigma_x^2 = \mathrm{Var}(X) = \sum_{i=1}^{n} (x_i - \mu)^2 p(x_i)$$

$$\sigma_x^2 \qquad 2$$

Variance is also given by

$$2 \qquad 2 \qquad ^2) = \sum_{i=1}^{n} x_i^2 p(x_i)$$

The non negative square root of the variance of a random variable is known as the standard deviation of the random variable. It is given by

$$\sigma_x = \sqrt{\mathrm{Var}(X)} = \sqrt{\sum_{i=1}^{n} (x_i - \mu)^2 p(x_i)}$$

Trials of a random experiment are called Bernoulli trials, if they satisfy the following conditions:

(ii) The trials should be independent.

(iv) The probability of success remains the same in each trial.

A binomial distribution with n -
cess in each trial as p). The probability function $P(X = x)$ or $P(x)$ of the binomial distribution is given by

$$P(x) = {}^nC_x q^{n-x} p^x \qquad x \qquad n \ (q = 1 - p)$$

BINOMIAL THEOREM

: A family of positive integers that occur as

We use the following formulae of combination to write the binomial

$${}^nC \ = 1 = {}^nC_n \ \text{and} \ {}^nC_r = \frac{n!}{r!(n-r)!} \qquad r \quad n$$

Pascal's Triangle
known as Pascal's Triangle.

Index	Coefficients					
0				$^0C_0$ (=1)		
1			$^1C_0$ (=1)		$^1C_1$ (=1)	
2		$^2C_0$ (=1)		$^2C_1$ (=2)		$^2C_2$ (=1)
3	$^3C_0$ (=1)	$^3C_1$ (=3)	$^3C_2$ (=3)	$^3C_3$ (=1)		
4	$^4C_0$ (=1)	$^4C_1$ (=4)	$^4C_2$ (=6)	$^4C_3$ (=4)	$^4C_4$ (=1)	
5	$^5C_0$ (=1)	$^5C_1$ (=5)	$^5C_2$ (=10)	$^5C_3$ (=10)	$^5C_4$ (=5)	$^5C_5$ (=1)

Binomial Theorem for Any Positive Integer n

$$(a+b)^n = {}^nC_0 a^n + {}^nC_1 a^{n-1}b + {}^nC_2 a^{n-2}b^2 + \ldots + {}^nC_{n-1}ab^{n-1} + {}^nC_n b^n$$

where ${}^nC_0, {}^nC_1, {}^nC_2, \ldots, {}^nC_n$ are called Binomial coefficients.

The notation $\sum\limits_{k=0}^{n} {}^nC_k\, a^{n-k}b^k$ for

$${}^nC_0 a^n b^0 + {}^nC_1 a^{n-1}b^1 + \ldots + {}^nC_r a^{n-r}b^r + \ldots + {}^nC_n a^{n-n}b^n,$$

where $b^0 = 1 = a^{n-n}$

Thus, the Binomial Theorem can also be written as:

$$(a+b)^n = \sum_{k=0}^{n} {}^nC_k\, a^{n-k}b^k$$

Properties of Binomial Expansion

(i) The sum of the indices of a and b is n in every term of the expansion.

(ii) There are $(n+1)$ terms in the expansion of $(a+b)^n$, the first and the last term being a^n and b^n respectively. If ${}^nC_x = {}^nC_y$, then either $x = y$ or $x + y = n$

(iii) The binomial coefficient in the expansion of $(a+b)^n$ which are equidistant from the beginning and the end are equal i.e. ${}^nC_r = {}^nC_{n-r}$.

Various Binomial Expansions

(i) $(x-y)^n = {}^nC_0 x^n - {}^nC_1 x^{n-1}y + {}^nC_2 x^{n-2} y^2 + \ldots + (-1)^n\, {}^nC_n y^n$

(ii) $(1+x)^n = {}^nC_0 + {}^nC_1 x + {}^nC_2 x^2 + {}^nC_3 x^3 + \ldots + {}^nC_n x^n$

(iii) $(1-x)^n = {}^nC_0 - {}^nC_1 x + {}^nC_2 x^2 - \ldots + (-1)^n\, {}^nC_n x^n$

Sum of Binomial Coefficients

Putting $x = 1$ in the expansion

$(1+x)^n = {}^nC_0 + {}^nC_1 x + {}^nC_2 x^2 + \ldots + {}^nC_n x^n$, we get,

$$2^n = {}^nC_0 + {}^nC_1 + {}^nC_2 + \ldots + {}^nC_n$$

(i) The $(r+1)^{th}$ term is known as the general term in the expansion of (   )^n. It is denoted by T_{r+1}

$$T_{r+1} = {}^nC_r \, a^{n-r} \, b^r$$

Similarly, the general term in the expansion of (   )^n is given as $T_{r+1} = {}^nC_r \, b^{n-r} \, a^r$. The terms are considered from the beginning.

(ii) If n is even, the middle term in the expansion of (   )^n is $\left(\dfrac{n}{2}+1\right)^{th}$ term.

(iii) If n is odd, there will be two middle terms in the expansion of (   )^n namely $\left(\dfrac{n+1}{2}\right)^{th}$ term and $\left(\dfrac{n+1}{2}+1\right)^{th}$ term.

(iv) In the expansion of $\left(x+\dfrac{1}{x}\right)^{2n}$, where x

$\left(\dfrac{2n+1+1}{2}\right)^{th}$, i.e., $(n+1)^{th}$ term, as $2n$ is even.

It is given by $2^n C_n x^n \left(\dfrac{1}{x}\right)^n = 2^n C_n$ (constant).

This term is called the *term independent* of x or the constant term

AVERAGE

(i) In a given data, average is given by
$$\text{Average} = \left(\frac{\text{Sum of observations}}{\text{Number of observations}}\right)$$

(ii) If the average of n_1 items is x_1, the average of n_2 items is x_2 and the average of n_3 items is x_3 then

$$\text{Total average} = \frac{n_1 x_1 + n_2 x_2 + n_3 x_3}{(n_1 + n_2 + n_3)}$$

$$n \text{ natural numbers} = \frac{(n+1)}{2}$$

$$n \text{ odd natural numbers} = n$$

$$n \text{ even natural numbers} = (n+1)$$

$$n \text{ natural numbers} = \frac{(n+1)(2n+1)}{6}$$

$$n \text{ natural numbers} = \frac{n(n+1)^2}{4}$$

$$n \text{ multiples of } x = \frac{x(n+1)}{2}$$

(i) Let the average of ages of p members of a family be q years. If a new member joins the family, then the new average of ages of all the members becomes r years, then

Age of the new member = $[r + p(r - q)]$ years.

(ii) Let the average of ages of p members of a family be q years. If one of the members leaves the family, then the new average of ages of all the members becomes r years, then

Age of the member leaving the family = [   ] years.

MEAN, MEDIAN, MODE

objective in mind, the data is said to be primary data.

Secondary data is the data collected by someone other than the user.

The mid point of a class interval is known as class mark. (It is assumed that the frequency of each class interval is centred around its mid point).

$$\text{Class Mark} = \frac{\text{Upper class limit} + \text{Lower class limit}}{2}$$

$$\text{Mean} = \frac{\text{Sum of observations}}{\text{Number of observations}}$$

If the frequency of a class is centred at its class mark, then the mean of the grouped data is determined by three methods.

(i) Direct Method

If x_1 $_2$ $_n$ are observations with frequencies f_1 $_2$ $_n$, respectively, then mean is given by

$$\bar{x} = \frac{f_1 x_1 + f_2 x_2 + \ldots + f_n x_n}{f_1 + f_2 + \ldots + f_n} \quad \text{or} \quad \bar{x} = \frac{\sum\limits_{i=1}^{n} f_i x_i}{\sum\limits_{i=1}^{n} f_i}$$

(ii) Assumed Mean Method

If $x_1, x_2, \ldots, x_n$ are observations with frequencies $f_1, f_2, \ldots, f_n$, respectively, a is the assumed mean and d_i is the deviation(difference between x_i and a), then mean is given by

$$\bar{x} = a + \frac{\sum f_i d_i}{\sum f_i}$$

(iii) Step Deviation Method

If $x_1, x_2, \ldots, x_n$ are observations with frequencies $f_1, f_2, \ldots, f_n$, respectively, a is the assumed mean and h is the class size, then mean is given by

$$\bar{x} = a + \left(\frac{\sum f_i u_i}{\sum f_i} \right) \times h \quad \text{where } u_i = \frac{x_i - a}{h}$$

Mode

Mode of Raw Data

The most frequently occurring observation is known as mode.

Modal Class

In a grouped frequency distribution, the class with the maximum frequency is known as modal class.

Mode of Grouped Data with Equal Class Size

If h is the class size, l the lower limit of the modal class, f_1 frequency of the modal class, f_0 frequency of the class preceding the modal class, f_2 frequency of the class succeeding the modal class, then mode is given by

$$\text{Mode} = l + \left(\frac{f_1 - f_0}{2 f_1 - f_0 - f_2} \right) \times h$$

Cumulative Frequency

The cumulative frequency of a class is the frequency obtained by adding the frequencies of all the classes preceding the given class.

- Cumulative frequency curve is known as an *ogive*.

Median

Median of Raw Data

The value of the middle most observation is known as median.

If n is an odd number, median = value of $\left(\frac{n+1}{2} \right)^{th}$ observation

If n is even, median = Mean of the value of $\left(\frac{n}{2} \right)^{th}$ and $\left(\frac{n}{2} + 1 \right)^{th}$ observation.

Median Class

If n is the number of observations, then the class whose cumulative frequency is greater than (and nearest to) $\dfrac{n}{2}$ is known as the median class.

Median of Grouped Data with Equal Class Size

If n is the number of observations, the lower limit of the median class, cf the cumulative frequency of the class preceding the median class, f frequency of the median class and h the class size, then median is given by

$$\text{Median} = +\left(\dfrac{\dfrac{n}{2} - cf}{f}\right) \times$$

x-coordinate of the point of intersection of two ogives gives the median of the grouped data.

3 Median = Mode + 2 Mean

Note: The mean, median and mode are called the measures of central tendency.

MEASURES OF DISPERSION

are known as measures of dispersion.

Range : The range of a data is the difference between the maximum and the minimum value.

If x_1 $_2$ $_n$ are n observations, then

$$\frac{1}{n}\sum_{i=1}^{n}|x_i - \bar{x}|, \text{ where } \bar{x} = \text{Mean}$$

$$\frac{1}{n}\sum_{i=1}^{n}|x_i - M|, \text{ where } M = \text{Median}$$

(a)

If x_1 $_2$ $_n$ are observations with frequencies f_1 $_2$ $_n$, respectively, then

$$\frac{1}{N}\sum_{i=1}^{n} f_i|x_i - \bar{x}| \text{ where } N = \sum_{i=1}^{n} f_i$$

(ii) Mean Deviation about median $= \dfrac{1}{N}\displaystyle\sum_{i=1}^{n} f_i |x_i - M|$ where $N = \displaystyle\sum_{i=1}^{n} f_i$

(b) *Continuous frequency distribution* : A continuous frequency distribution is a series in which the data are classified into different class-intervals without gaps alongwith their respective frequencies.

If $x_1, x_2, \ldots, x_n$ are observations with frequencies $f_1, f_2, \ldots, f_n$, respectively, a is the assumed mean and h is the class size, then Mean by step-deviation

$$(\bar{x}) = a + \dfrac{\displaystyle\sum_{i=1}^{n} f_i d_i}{N} \times h$$

where $d_i = \dfrac{x_i - a}{h}$ and $N = \displaystyle\sum_{i=1}^{n} f_i$

If N is the sum of frequencies, l, C, f and h are respectively the lower limit , the cumulative frequency of the class just preceding the median class(the class interval whose cumulative frequency is just greater than or equal to $\dfrac{N}{2}$) , frequency and the width of the median class, then

$$\text{Median} = l + \dfrac{\dfrac{N}{2} - C}{f} \times h$$

Variance
Mean of the squares of the deviations from mean is called the variance. Variance of n observations $x_1, x_2, \ldots, x_n$ is

$$\sigma^2 = \dfrac{1}{n}\sum_{i=1}^{n}(x_i - \bar{x})^2$$

Standard Deviation
Positive square root of the variance is called standard deviation.

$$\sigma = \sqrt{\dfrac{1}{n}\sum_{i=1}^{n}(x_i - \bar{x})^2}$$

Standard Deviation of a Discrete Frequency Distribution

If $x_1, x_2, \ldots, x_n$ are observations with frequencies $f_1, f_2, \ldots, f_n$, then

$$\sigma = \sqrt{\dfrac{1}{N}\sum_{i=1}^{n} f_i(x_i - \bar{x})^2} \ , \text{ where } N = \sum_{i=1}^{n} f_i$$

If there is a frequency distribution of n
its mid-point x_i with frequency f_i then

$$\sigma = \frac{1}{N}\sqrt{N\sum_{i=1}^{n}f_i x_i^2 - \left(\sum_{i=1}^{n}f_i x_i\right)^2} \ , \ \text{where } N = \sum_{i=1}^{n}f_i$$

If $x_1, \ _2 \quad _n$ are observations with frequencies $f_1, \ _2 \qquad _n,$ A the
assumed mean, h the class size and y_i the step deviation then,

$$\sigma = \frac{h}{N}\sqrt{N\sum_{i=1}^{n}f_i y_i^2 - \left(\sum_{i=1}^{n}f_i y_i\right)^2} \ , \ \text{where } \ y_i = \frac{x_i - A}{h} \ , \ N = \sum_{i=1}^{n}f_i$$

The measure of variability which is independent of units is called

$$\frac{\sigma}{x}\times \qquad , \ \bar{x} \neq \quad , \text{ where } \bar{x} = \text{mean and}$$

σ = standard deviation
For series with equal means, the series with lesser standard deviation
is more consistent or less scattered.

SETS

If a is an element of set A, we write a A and if a is not an element
of A, we write a A.

(i)   : In roster form, all the elements of a set
are listed, they are separated by commas and are enclosed within

not important.

form.

(ii) *Set-builder form* : In set-builder form, all the elements of a set possess a single common property which is not possessed by any element outside the set.

Common Symbols of Some Sets

- N: The set of all natural numbers
- Z: The set of all integers
- Q: The set of all rational numbers
- T: The set of all irrational numbers
- R: The set of real numbers
- Z^+: The set of positive integers
- Q^+: The set of positive rational numbers
- R^+: The set of positive real numbers
- U: The universal set

Empty Set : A set which does not contain any element is called an empty set or null set or void set.

Singleton Set : If a set has only one element, it is called a singleton set.

Finite and Infinite Set : A set which is empty or consists of a definite number of elements is called a finite set, otherwise, the set is called an infinite set.

- An infinite set cannot be written in the roster form.

Equality of Sets : Two sets A and B are said to be equal if they have exactly the same elements.

- A set does not change if one or more elements are repeated.

Subset : A set A is said to be subset of a set B, if every element of A is also an element of B.

- $A \subset B$ if $a \in A \Rightarrow a \in B$
- $A \subset B$ and $B \subset A \Leftrightarrow A = B$
- Every set is a subset of itself.
- Null set is a subset of every set.
- If set A is a subset of set B and $A \neq B$, then A is called a proper subset of B and B is called superset of A.
- $N \subset Z \subset Q, Q \subset R, T \subset R, N \not\subset T$

Power Set : A power set of a set A is collection of all subsets of A. It is denoted by P(A).

If A is a set with $n(A) = m$, then $n[P(A)] = 2^m$ where $n(A)$ denotes the number of elements in set A.

Intervals as Subsets of R

Open Interval

The set of real numbers $\{ y : a < y < b \}$, where $a, b \in$ R and $a < b$ is called an open interval and is denoted by (a, b).

All the points between a and b belong to the open interval (a, b) but a, b themselves do not belong to this interval.

Closed Interval

The interval which contains the end points also is called closed interval and is denoted by $[a, b]$. Thus $[a, b] = \{x : a \leq x \leq b\}$ where $a, b \in$ R

Half open, Half closed

(i) $[a, b) = \{x : a \leq x < b\}$ is an open interval from a to b, including a but excluding b.

(ii) $(a, b] = \{x : a < x \leq b\}$ is an open interval from a to b including b but excluding a.

The number $(b - a)$ is called the length of any of the intervals $(a, b), [a, b], [a, b)$ or $(a, b]$.

Intervals on the Number Line

(a,b)	$[a,b]$	$[a,b)$	$(a,b]$

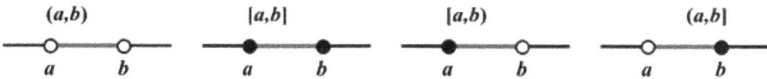

Union of Sets: The union of two sets A and B is the set of all those elements which are either in A or in B. The symbol $\cup$ is used to represent union.

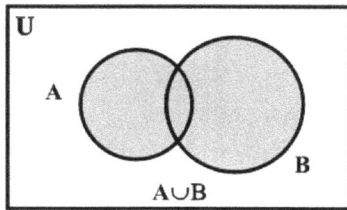

A∪B

Properties of Union

(i)   A∪B = B∪A (Commutative Law)

(ii) (A∪B) ∪ C = A∪(B∪C) (Associative law)

(iii) A ∪ φ = A (Law of identity element, φ is the identity of ∪)

(iv) A ∪ A = A (Idempotent law)

(v)   U ∪ A = U (Law of U)

Intersection of Sets: The intersection of two sets A and B is the set of all elements which are common. The symbol ∩ is used to represent intersection of sets.

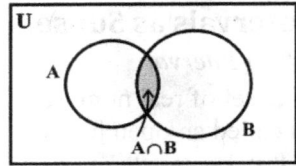

A∩B

Properties of Intersection

(i) $A \cap B = B \cap A$ (Commutative law)

(ii) $(A \cap B) \cap C = A \cap (B \cap C)$ (Associative law)

(iii) $\phi \cap A = \phi$, $U \cap A = A$ (Law of ϕ and U)

(iv) $A \cap A = A$ (Idempotent law)

(v) $A \cap (B \cup C) = (A \cap B) \cup (A \cap C)$ (Distributive law)

Disjoint Set : If A and B are two sets such that $A \cap B = \varphi$ then A and B are called disjoint sets.

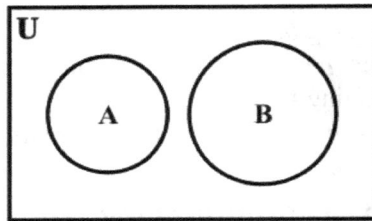

Difference of Sets : The difference of two sets A and B in this order is the set of elements which belong to A but not to B.

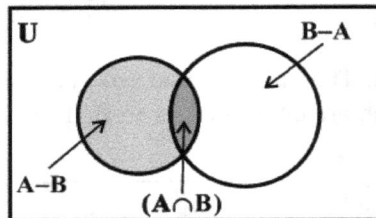

Complement of a Set : The complement of a subset A of universal set U is the set of all elements of U which are not the elements of A.

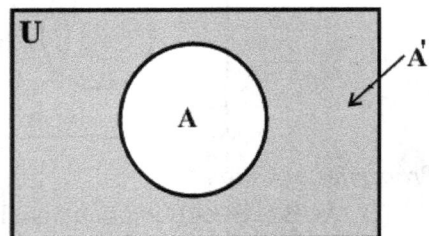

If A is a subset of universal set U, then its compliment A' is also a subset of U.

Properties of Complement

(i) For any set A, $(A')' = A$ (Law of double complement)

(ii) For any two sets A and B, $(A \cup B)' = A' \cap B'$ and $(A \cap B)' = A' \cup B'$ (De Morgan's Law)

(iii) A   (Complement Law)

(iv)   '= U and U' =

, then

$n(A$ $n(A) + n$

, then

$n(A$ $n(A) + n$ n

$n(A$ $C) = n(A) + n$

$n(C) - n$ n n n

RELATION, FUNCTION AND BINARY OPERATION

Ordered pair : A pair of elements grouped together in a particular order is known as an ordered pair.

ments are equal i.e. If   , then $a = x$ and   and if
$a = x$ and   then

): a A,

is called

an ordered triplet.

=

x and the second element y of the ordered

A relation may be represented algebraically either in the Roster form or in the Set-builder form.
An arrow diagram is used to represent a relation.
A relation R from A to A is known as a relation on A.
If there are x elements in A and y
be xy $n(A) = x$ and n y, then

$n(A \times B) = xy$ and the total number of relations is 2^{xy}.

Image : The image of an element x under a relation R is given by y, where $(x, y) \in R$,

Domain : The domain of R is the set of all first elements of the ordered pairs in a relation R from a set A to a set B.

Range : The range of R is the set of all second elements of the ordered pairs in a relation R from a set A to a set B. The whole set B is called the co-domain of the relation R.

Types of Relation

Empty Relation
A relation R in a set A is called empty relation, if no element of A is related to any element of A, i.e., $R = \phi \subset A \times A$

Universal Relation
A relation R in a set A is called universal relation if each element of A is related to every element of A, i.e., $R = A \times A$

Reflexive, Symmetric and Transitive Relation
A relation R in a set A is called
(i)   reflexive , if $(a, a) \in R$, for every $a \in A$,
(ii) symmetric, if $(a_1, a_2) \in R$ implies that $(a_2, a_1) \in R$, for all $a_1, a_2 \in A$
(iii) transitive , if $(a_1, a_2) \in R$ and $(a_2, a_3) \in R$ implies that $(a_1, a_3) \in R$, for all $a_1, a_2, a_3 \in A$

Equivalence Relation
A relation R in a set A is said to be an equivalence relation if R is reflexive, symmetric and transitive.

Equivalence Class
If R is an arbitrary equivalence relation in an arbitrary set X and R divides X into mutually disjoint subsets A_i, then A_i are called partitions or subdivisions of X satisfying:
(i)   all elements of A_i are related to each other, for all i
(ii) no element of A_i is related to any element of A_j, $i \neq j$
(iii) $\cup A_j = X$ and $A_i \cap A_j = \phi$, $i \neq j$
      The subsets A_i are called equivalence classes

Function
A function f from a set A to a set B is a specific type of relation for which every element x of set A has one and only one image y in set B.
If $f: A \rightarrow B$ and $(x,y) \in f$, where $f(x) = y$, then
(i)   A is the domain and B is the codomain of f.
(ii) y is called the image of x under f and x is called the pre-image of y.

Mathematics Formulae

(iii) The range of the function is the set of images.

Real Function

A function which has either R or one of its subsets as its range is called a real valued function. If its domain is also either R or a subset of R, it is called a real function.

Explicit and Implicit Function

y is an *explicit function* of *x* if the relationship between *x* and *y* is expressed in a way that it is easy to solve for *y* *i.e.* one variable is defined in terms of the other variable.

y is an *implicit function* of *x* if the relationship between *x* and *y* is expressed in a way that it is not easy to solve for *y*.

Special Functions

Identity Function

If R is a real number, then the real valued function $f: R \rightarrow R$, where $y = f(x) = x$ for each $x \in R$ is known as an identity function.

- The graph of an identity function is a straight line passing through the origin.

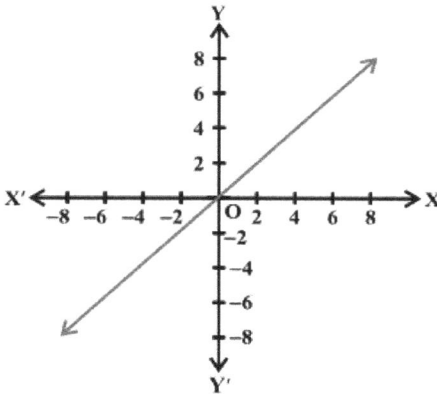

- The domain and range of identity function is R.

Constant Function

If R is a real number, then the function $f: R \rightarrow R$, where $y = f(x) = c$ for each $x \in R$ and c a constant is known as a constant function.

- The graph of a constant function is a horizontal line (parallel to *x* axis).

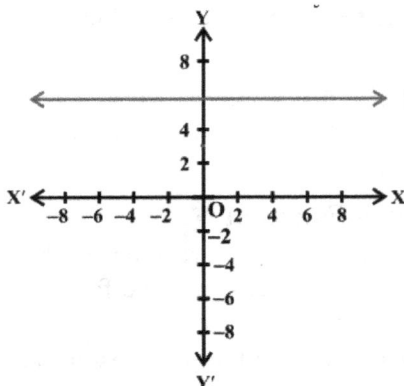

- The domain of identity function is R and range is {c}.

Polynomial Function

If R is a real number, then $f: R \rightarrow R$, such that
$$y = f(x) = a_n x^n + a_{n-1} x^{n-1} + \ldots + a_2 x^2 + a_1 x + a_0;$$
where n is a non negative integer, $a_n \neq 0$ and $a_n, a_1, a_2, \ldots, a_n \in R$ is known as a polynomial function.

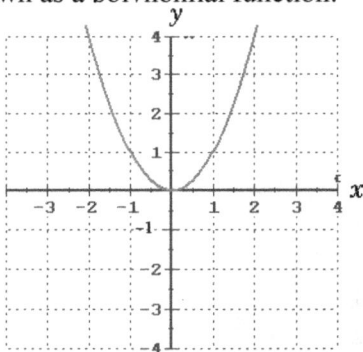

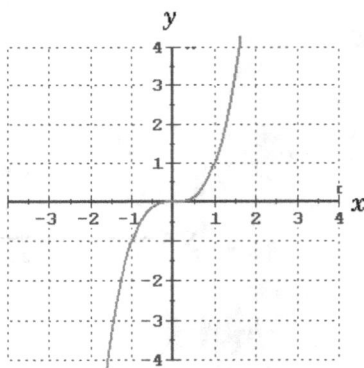

- The graph of a polynomial function has different shapes depending on the degree of the polynomial.

Rational Function

The functions of the type $\dfrac{f(x)}{g(x)}$, where $f(x)$ and $g(x)$ are polynomial functions of x defined in a domain, and $g(x) \neq 0$ are called rational function.

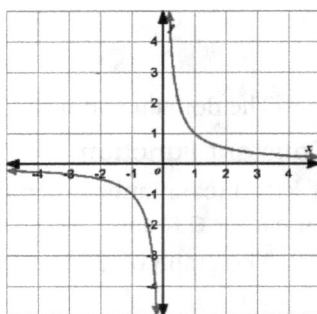

Modulus Function

If R is a real number, then the function
$f: R \rightarrow R$, where $y = f(x) = |x|$
for each $x \in R$ is known as a modulus function.

$$f(x) = \begin{cases} x, x \geq 0 \\ -x, x < 0 \end{cases}$$

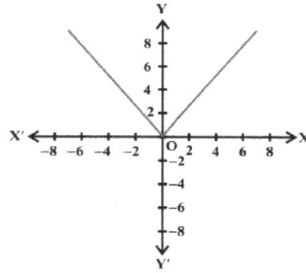

Signum Function

If R is a real number, then the function
$f: R \rightarrow R$, where the function

$$y = f(x) = \begin{cases} -1 \text{ if } x < 0 \\ 0 \text{ if } x = 0 \\ 1 \text{ if } x > 0 \end{cases}$$

is known as signum function.

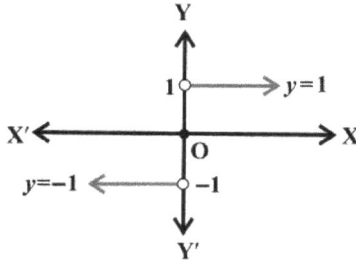

Exponential Function

The function $y = f(x) = b^x$ with positive base $b > 1$ is known as the exponential function.

Properties of exponential function

(i) Domain of the exponential function is the set of all real numbers (R).
(ii) Range of the exponential function is the set of all positive real numbers (R^+).
(iii) The point (0, 1) always lies on the graph of the exponential function.
(iv) Exponential function is an increasing function.
(v) For very large negative values of x, the graph of the exponential function approaches x-axis in the second quadrant but never meets it.

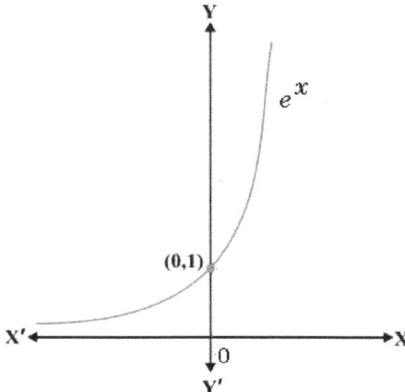

Note:

Exponential function with base 10 is called the *common exponential function.*

Exponential function with base *e* is called natural *exponential function.*

Logarithmic Function

The function defined by $\log_b$: $R^+ \to R$, $x \to log_b x = y$ if $b^y = x$ is called logarithmic function.

Salient features of logarithmic function

(i) Domain of the logarithmic function is the set of all positive real numbers (R^+).

(ii) Range of the logarithmic function is the set of all real numbers (R).

(iii) The point $(1, 0)$ always lies on the graph of the logarithmic function.

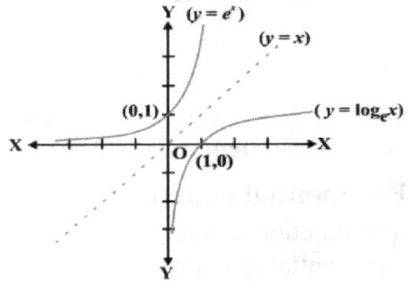

(iv) Logarithmic function is an increasing function.

(v) For *x* very close to zero, the graph of the logarithmic function approaches *y*-axis in the fourth quadrant but never meets it.

(vi) The graph of $y = e^x$ and $y = log_e x$ are the mirror images of each other reflected at the line $y = x$.

Note:

Logarithmic function with base(*b*) 10 is called the *common logarithmic function.*

Logarithmic function with base *e* is called natural *logarithmic function.* It is generally represented by *ln*.

Greatest Integer Function

If R is a real number, then the function *f*: $R \to R$, defined by $f(x) = [x]$, $x \in R$ where *f(x)* is the greatest integer less than or equal to *x* is known as the greatest integer function.

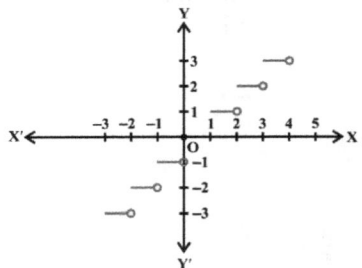

- The domain of greatest integer function is (-infinity, infinity).
- The range of greatest integer function is integers.

Types of Functions
Injective Function
A function $f\colon X \to Y$ is injective or one-one if $f(x_1) = f(x_2)$ $\Rightarrow x_1 = x_2, \forall\, x_1, x_2 \in X$. Otherwise the function is called many one.

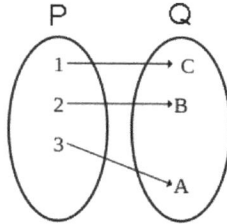

Surjective Function
A function $f\colon X \to Y$
is surjective or onto if for every $y \in Y$, $\exists\, x \in X$ such that $f(x) = y$.

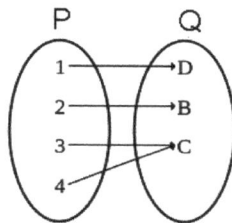

Bijective Function
A function $f\colon X \to Y$ is bijective, if f is both one-one and onto.

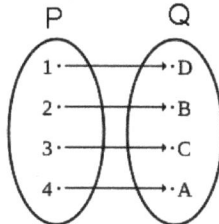

Composition of f and g
The composition of functions $f\colon A \to B$ and $g\colon B \to C$ is the function $gof\colon A \to C$ given by $gof(x) = g(f(x))\ \forall\, x \in A$.

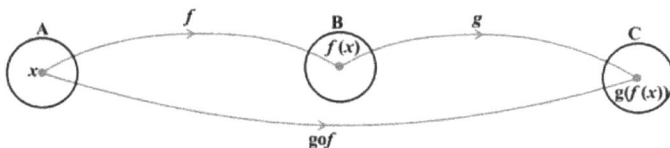

Properties of Composition

(i) If $f: X \to Y$, $g: Y \to Z$ and $h: Z \to S$ are functions, then
$$ho(gof) = (hog)of$$

(ii) Let $f: X \to Y$ and $g: Y \to Z$ be two invertible functions. Then gof is also invertible with $(gof)^{-1} = f^{-1}og^{-1}$

Inverse of a Function

A function $f: X \to Y$ is invertible if $\exists$ a function $g: Y \to X$ such that $gof = I_X$ and $fog = I_Y$. The function g is called the inverse of f. It is denoted by f^{-1}.

A function $f: X \to Y$ is invertible if and only if f is one-one and onto.

Properties of Functions

Let $f: X \to R$ and $g: X \to R$ be any two real functions where X is a subset of R, then

(i) $(f + g): X \to R$ is defined by $(f + g)(x) = f(x) + g(x)$ for all $x \in R$

(ii) $(f - g): X \to R$ is defined by $(f - g)(x) = f(x) - g(x)$ for all $x \in R$

(iii) $(kf)(x) = kf(x)$ for all $x \in R$ and k a scalar

(iv) $(fg)(x) = f(x)\, g(x)$ for all $x \in R$

(v) $\left(\dfrac{f}{g}\right)(x) = \dfrac{f(x)}{g(x)}$, provided $g(x) \neq 0$, $x \in X$

Binary Operation

A binary operation $*$ on a set A is a function $*: A \times A \to A$. We represent $* \, (a, b)$ by $a * b$.

Properties of Binary Operation

Commutative Property

A binary operation $*$ on the set X is called commutative, if $a * b = b * a$, for every $a, b \in X$.

Associative Property

A binary operation $* : A \times A \to A$ is said to be associative if $(a * b) * c = a * (b * c)$, $\forall\, a, b, c \in A$.

Identity element

Given a binary operation $*: A \times A \to A$, an element $e \in A$, if it exists, is called identity for the operation $*$, if $a * e = a = e * a$. $\forall\, a \in A$.

Inverse

Given a binary operation $*: A \times A \to A$ with the identity element e in A, an element $a \in A$ is said to be invertible with respect to the operation $*$, if there exists an element b in A such that $a * b = e = b * a$ and b is called the inverse of a and is denoted by a^{-1}.

LINEAR PROGRAMMING

(maximum or minimum) of a linear function of several variables (called objective function) subject to the conditions that the variables are non-negative and satisfy a set of linear inequalities (called *constraints*).

Objective function: Linear function $Z =$ (are constants), which has to be maximised or minimized is called a linear objective function. Variables x and y are called They are non-negative.

Constraints: The restrictions or linear inequalities or equations on the variables of a linear programming problem are called constraints. The conditions are called non-negative restrictions.

Optimisation problem: A problem which seeks to maximise or minimise a linear function subject to certain constraints as determined by a set of linear inequalities is called an optimisation problem.

(ii) Manufacturing problems

(iii)Transportation problems

The common region determined by all the constraints including the non-negative constraints of a linear programming problem is called the feasible region (or solution region) for the problem.

-

sent feasible solutions of the constraints.

Any point in the feasible region that gives the optimal value (maximum or minimum) of the objective function is called an optimal solution.

(i) Let R be the feasible region (convex polygon) for a linear programming problem and let $Z =$ be the objective function. When Z has an optimal value (maximum or minimum), where the variables x and y are subject to constraints described by linear inequalities, this optimal value must occur at a corner point (vertex) of the feasible region.

(ii) Let R be the feasible region for a linear programming problem, and let $Z = ax + by$ be the objective function.

(a) If R is bound, then the objective function Z has both a maximum and a minimum value on R and each of these occurs at a corner point (vertex) of R.

(b) If the feasible region is unbound, then a maximum or a minimum may not exist, if it exists, it must occur at a corner point of R.

Corner Point Method

(i) Find the feasible region of the linear programming problem and determine its corner points (vertices) either by solving the two equations of the lines intersecting at that point or by inspection.

(ii) Evaluate the objective function $Z = ax + by$ at each corner point. Let M and m respectively be the largest and smallest values at these points.

(iii) If the feasible region is bound, M and m respectively are the maximum and minimum values of the objective function.

(iv) If the feasible region is unbound, then

(a) M is the maximum value of the objective function, if the open half plane determined by $ax + by > M$ has no point in common with the feasible region. Otherwise, the objective function has no maximum value.

(b) m is the minimum value of the objective function, if the open half plane determined by $ax + by < m$ has no point in common with the feasible region. Otherwise, the objective function has no minimum value.

If two corner points of the feasible region are both optimal solutions of the same type, i.e., both produce the same maximum or minimum, then any point on the line segment joining these two points is also an optimal solution of the same type.

Data Interpretation

lection of data is followed by its analysis and interpretation.

assigned to the collected information followed by the determination

sectors in a circle. The angle of a sector is proportional to the frequency of the data.

The formula to determine the angle of a sector is:

$$\text{Angle of sector} = \frac{\text{Frequency of data}}{\text{Total frequency}} \times \quad °$$

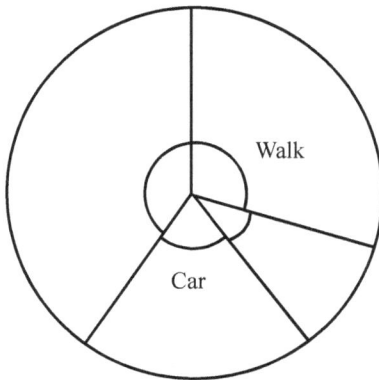

Walk

Car

graphical display of data using rectangular bars of different heights. The height of the bar is proportional to the value it represents. The bars can be plotted vertically or horizontally.

Number of students

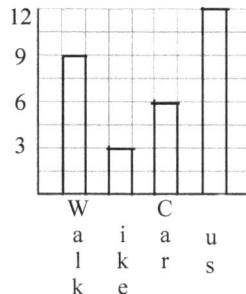

12
9
6
3

W C
a i a u
l k r s
k e

Line Graph

A line graph is a graph that uses line segments to connect points that represent the value of the variables.

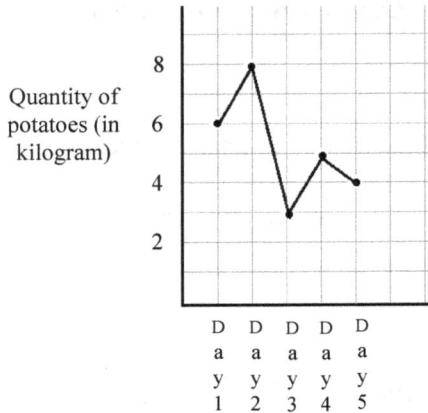

Quantity of potatoes (in kilogram)

D	D	D	D	D
a	a	a	a	a
y	y	y	y	y
1	2	3	4	5

Histogram

A histogram is the representation of a frequency distribution by means of rectangles whose widths represent class interval and whose areas are proportional to the corresponding frequencies.

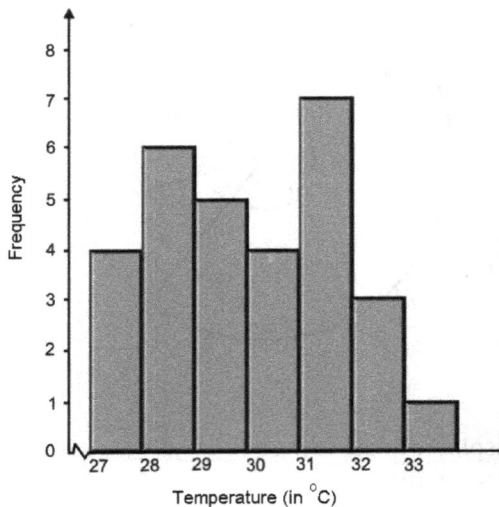

Temperature (in °C)

Frequency Polygon

A line graph drawn by joining all the mid points of the tops of the bars of the histogram is known as a frequency polygon.

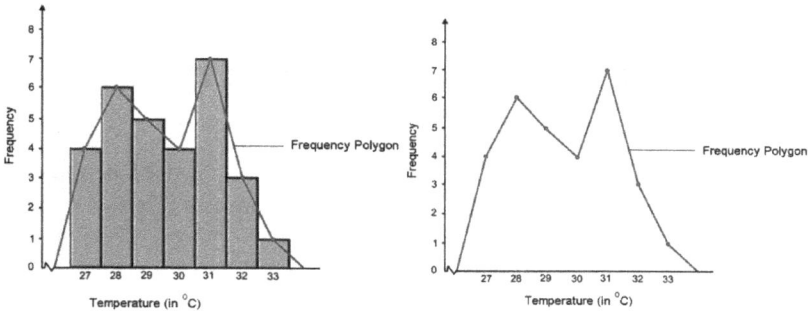

Note: In order to save time in data interpretation questions visual estimation, approximation and reasoning can be used instead of actual calculation.

Dynamics Formulae

MOTION IN A STRAIGHT LINE

The branch of mechanics that deals with the motion of a body or system of bodies under the action of forces from outside the system

Motion : A body is said to be in motion if it changes its position with

Rest : A body is said to be at rest if it does not change its position with respect to a reference point.

A physical quantity which has only magnitude is called a *quantity*.
A physical quantity which has both magnitude and direction is called a *vector quantity*.

The actual length of the path covered by the body irrespective of the direction is called the *distance*. It is a scalar quantity. The SI unit of distance is metre.

                    is the shortest distance (straight distance) between the

quantity. The SI unit of displacement is metre.

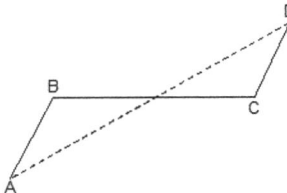

In the given diagram,

Displacement = The shortest path between A and D

= AD along the direction A to D

Speed and Velocity

Speed is the rate of change of position of an object. It is a scalar quantity (i.e. it has only magnitude and no direction). The SI unit of speed is m/s.

Velocity is the rate of change of position of an object in a particular direction. It is a vector quantity (i.e. it has both magnitude and direction). The SI unit of velocity is m/s.

Let a particle move from a point O along the direction OX. Let the

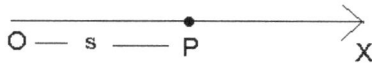

$$O \longmapsto s \longmapsto P \longrightarrow X$$

displacement of the particle be OP = s in time t. Then,

Velocity $= \dfrac{ds}{dt}$

Uniform Velocity

A body is said to have a uniform velocity if it travels in a straight line (in a particular direction) and covers equal distances in equal intervals of time.

Uniform Velocity = Constant $\dfrac{ds}{dt}$ throughout the interval

Average velocity

If the velocity of a body changes continuously at a uniform rate, the arithmetic mean of the initial and final velocities over a given period of time is called its average velocity.

Average velocity $= \dfrac{\text{Initial velocity} + \text{Final velocity}}{2}$ or $v_{av} = \dfrac{u+v}{2}$

Distance = Average velocity × Time

Relative Velocity of Two Bodies Moving Along a Straight Line

Let the velocities of two bodies P and Q at any instant be u and u' respectively.

Let s and s' be the distance of P and Q respectively from a fixed point O of the straight line.

Velocity of Q relative to P = Rate of change of the distance

PQ $= \frac{d}{dt}(s'-s) = \frac{ds'}{dt} - \frac{ds}{dt} = u' - u$

Or

Velocity of Q relative to P = Velocity of Q + Reversed velocity of P

Acceleration

The rate of change of velocity is called acceleration. The SI unit of acceleration is m/s². It is given by

$$\frac{dv}{dt} \text{ or } \frac{d^2s}{dt^2} \text{ or } v\frac{dv}{ds}$$

Uniform Acceleration

An object has a uniform acceleration if it travels in a straight line and its velocity increases or decreases by equal amounts in equal intervals of time.

Retardation

Negative acceleration is called retardation. In this case the velocity of a body decreases with time i.e. the final velocity is less than the initial velocity.

Equations of Motion

Relationships between initial velocity (u), final velocity (v), distance (s), acceleration (a), and time taken (t), in the case of a moving object, are called equations of motion.

First Equation of Motion

Let s be the displacement of a particle in time t. Then the acceleration is given by

$$\frac{d^2s}{dt^2} = a$$

Integrating both sides with respect to t we get, $\frac{ds}{dt} = at + c$ where c is the constant of integration.

At time $t = 0$, $\frac{ds}{dt} = u$, hence $c = u$ Therefore, $\frac{ds}{dt} = at + u$

or $v = u + at$ *(Velocity–Time Relation)*

Second Equation of Motion

$\frac{ds}{dt} = at + u$ (From first equation of motion)

Integrating both sides with respect to t we get, $s = \frac{1}{2}at^2 + ut + k$

where k is the constant of integration
At time $t = 0$, $s = 0$, hence $k = 0$

Therefore, $s = \frac{1}{2}at^2 + ut$ Or $s = ut + \frac{1}{2}at^2$ (*Position Time Relation*)

Third Equation of Motion

$v\frac{dv}{ds} = a$ (By definition of acceleration)

Integrating both sides with respect to s we get, $\frac{1}{2}v^2 = as + c$
where c is the constant of integration. Initially when $s = 0$, $v = u$
and $\frac{1}{2}u^2 = c$

Therefore, $\frac{1}{2}v^2 = as + \frac{1}{2}u^2$

Or $\frac{1}{2}v^2 - \frac{1}{2}u^2 = as$

Or $v^2 - u^2 = 2as$
Or $v^2 = u^2 + 2as$ *(Position Velocity Relation)*

Note:
- When a body starts from rest initial velocity u is taken as zero.
- When a body comes to rest the final velocity v is taken as zero.
- When a body moves with constant velocity acceleration a is zero.

Equations of Motion When a Body Starts From Rest

If a body starts from rest initial velocity is zero ($u = 0$). Hence the equations of motion are:

(i) $v = at$ *(Velocity-Time Relation)*

(ii) $s = \frac{1}{2}at^2$ *(Position Time Relation)*

(iii) $v^2 = 2as$ *(Position Velocity Relation)*

The above three equations of motion are equations of a body moving along a straight line with constant acceleration.

COMPOSITION OF VELOCITY

A body may have two or more displacements simultaneously in different directions. This is known as co-existence of displacement.

A body may have two or more velocities simultaneously in different directions. This is known as co-existence of velocity.

If a body has two displacements represented by the two sides OA and

sented by the diagonal OC.

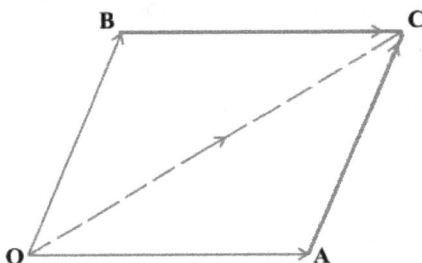

Parallelogram law of velocity states that if two velocities can be represented both in magnitude and direction by two adjacent sides of a parallelogram drawn from the same point then their resultant is represented both in magnitude and direction on the same scale by the diagonal passing through the same point.

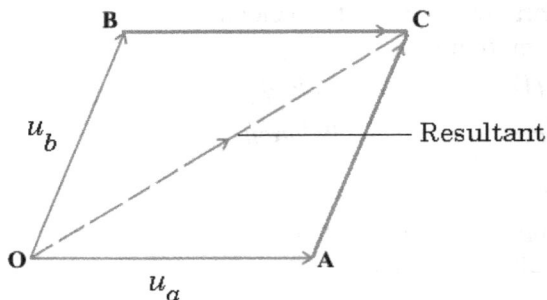

Triangle law of velocity states that if two velocities can be represented both in magnitude and direction by two sides of a triangle taken in the same order then their resultant is represented both in magnitude and direction by the third side of the triangle taken in the reverse order (opposite direction).

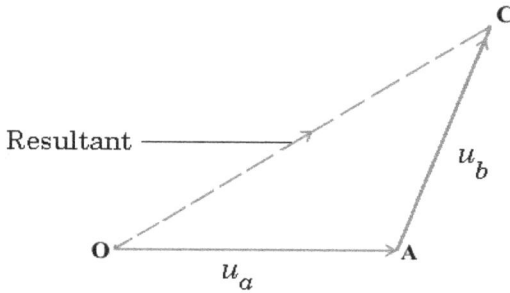

Splitting of a velocity into its components is known as resolution of velocity.

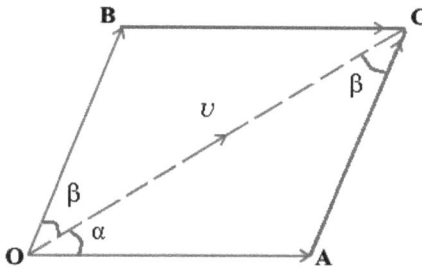

v and let the velocity

v

$$= \frac{v \sin \beta}{\mathrm{Sin}\,(\alpha + \beta)} \qquad = \frac{v\,\mathrm{Sin}\,\alpha}{\mathrm{Sin}\,(\alpha + \beta)}$$

CIRCULAR MOTION

When a body moves along a circular path in such a way that the direction of motion at any point is given by the tangent drawn at that point, its motion is called circular motion.

Angular Displacement

When the body moves in a circle along the circumference, the angle described by the line joining the object to the centre of the circle, is called its angular displacement. In the given figure, angular displacement = θ. The SI unit of angular displacement is radian.

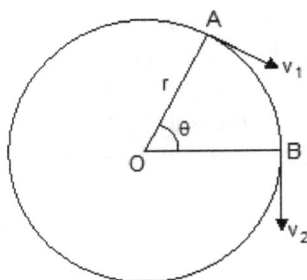

Angular Velocity

The angular velocity is defined as the rate of change of the angular displacement with time. It is denoted by ω (omega) and is given by,

$$\omega = \frac{d\theta}{dt}$$

The SI unit of angular velocity is radians/second.

Angular Acceleration

The rate of change of angular velocity is called angular acceleration. It is given by,

Angular acceleration $= \dfrac{d\omega}{dt} = \dfrac{d}{dt}\left(\dfrac{d\theta}{dt}\right) = \dfrac{d^2\theta}{dt^2}$

The SI unit of angular acceleration is radians/second^2.

Relation Between Linear Velocity and Angular Velocity

Let a particle move from point A to point B along a circular path covering a linear distance s. Let the radius of the circle be r and the angular displacement be θ then,

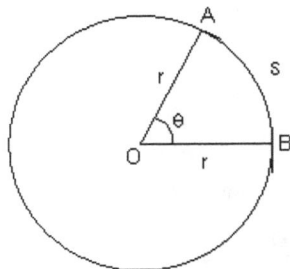

$$\text{Angle} = \frac{\text{Arc}}{\text{Radius}}$$

Or, $\theta = \dfrac{s}{r}$ Or $s = r\,\theta$

Differentiating both sides with respect to time, we get $\dfrac{ds}{dt} = \dfrac{d}{dt}(r\theta)$

Since radius is constant, $\dfrac{ds}{dt} = r\dfrac{d\theta}{dt}$

Or $v = r\omega$ [Since $v = \dfrac{ds}{dt}$ and $\omega = \dfrac{d\theta}{dt}$]

MOTION UNDER GRAVITY

The force of attraction between any two bodies in the universe is known as gravitation.

The force of attraction between the earth and any object lying on its surface is known as gravity.

alone, we say that the objects are in free fall.

The acceleration acquired by a body due to the earth's gravitational pull on it is known as acceleration due to gravity. It is denoted by g. The value of g ^{2}.

As 'g' is constant near the earth, all the equations for the uniformly accelerated motion of objects become valid with acceleration 'a' replaced by 'g' and distance 's' replaced by height 'h'.

(i) $v = u + gt$

(ii) $h = ut + \dfrac{1}{2}gt^2$

(iii) $v^2 = u^2 + 2gh$

where

u = Initial velocity
v = Final velocity
h = Height
t = Time

If a body falls from rest initial velocity is zero ($u = 0$). Hence, the equations of motion reduces to:

(i) $v = gt$

(ii) $h = \dfrac{1}{2}gt^2$

(iii) $v^2 = 2gh$

When a body is thrown upwards, the acceleration is taken as negative; hence the equations of motion reduces to

(i) $v = u - gt$

(ii) $h = ut - \dfrac{1}{2}gt^2$

(iii) $v^2 = u^2 - 2gh$

Time of Ascent and Maximum Height

v

Using $v = u - gt$ we get, Time of ascent $= t = \dfrac{u}{g}$

Using $v^2 = u^2 - 2gh$ we get,

Maximum height $= h = \dfrac{u^2}{2g}$

The instant when the body starts h

Hence, by using $h = ut - \dfrac{1}{2}gt^2$ we get $t = 0$ or $t = \dfrac{2u}{g}$

In other words, $t = 0$ is the instant when the body starts and $t = \dfrac{2u}{g}$ is the instant when the body returns to the starting point.

$$= \dfrac{2u}{g}$$

and Time of descent = Time of ascent $= \dfrac{u}{g}$

NEWTON'S LAWS OF MOTION

A push or a pull which changes or tends to change the state of rest or of uniform motion or direction of motion of a body is known as force. Its SI unit is Newton.

An object at rest or in uniform motion will remain at rest or in uniform motion unless an unbalanced force acts on it. This law is also called the law of inertia.

Newton's Second Law of Motion

Momentum

It is a measure of the quantity of motion in any object. Its SI unit is kg m/s. It is given by

Momentum = Mass × Velocity

Rate of Change of Momentum

If a body has mass m, initial velocity u, final velocity v in time t, then

Rate of change of momentum $= \dfrac{m \times (v - u)}{t}$

Statement of Second Law of Motion

Newton's Second Law of Motion states that the rate of change of momentum of a body is proportional to the unbalanced force acting on it and takes place in the direction of the force.

If a force F acts on a body of mass m and velocity v, then

$F = k \dfrac{d}{dt}(mv)$, where k is the constant of proportionality.

Since the mass is constant, $F = km \dfrac{dv}{dt} = kma$

If F = 1 Newton, $m = 1$kg, $a = 1$m/s^2, then $k = 1$.

Hence, F $= ma$

Or Force = mass × acceleration

When force (F) = 0, $\dfrac{d}{dt}(mv) = 0$, therefore momentum is constant.

Hence, the body continues to move with constant momentum when no external force acts on it.

Weight

The force with which an object is attracted towards the earth is known as weight of the object. The SI unit of weight is Newton (kgm/s^2).

Weight = Mass × Acceleration due to gravity

Or W $= m \times g$

Newton's Third Law of Motion

Whenever two bodies interact, the force exerted by the first body on the second (called action) is equal and opposite to that exerted by the second body on the first body (called reaction). This law may also be stated as "To every action there is an equal and opposite reaction."

PROJECTILE MOTION

A form of motion in which an object or a particle (called a projectile) is thrown near the surface of the earth and it moves along a curved path under the action of gravity is known as projectile motion. The object is projected in a direction oblique to the direction of gravity.

Projectile motion is a two dimensional motion – one along the x-axis(horizontal motion) and the other along the y-axis (vertical motion).

Horizontal motion and vertical motion are independent of each other.

A body can be projected in two ways:

(i)   : When the body has an initial velocity in the horizontal direction only, it is known as horizontal projection.

(ii)   : When the body is thrown with an initial velocity at an angle to the horizontal direction, it is known as angular projection.

Horizontal Projection

Let a body be thrown from the origin with an initial velocity u along the horizontal direction.

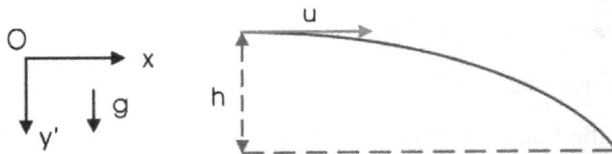

Along x axis	Along y axis
Component of initial velocity along x axis is $u_x = u$	Component of initial velocity along y axis is $u_y = 0$
Acceleration along x axis is a_x	Acceleration along y axis is $a_y = g$
Component of velocity along x axis at any instant t is $v_x = u_x + a_x t$ $v_x = u + 0$ $v_x = u$	Component of velocity along y axis at any instant t is $v_y = u_y + a_y t$ $v_y = 0 + gt$ $v_y = gt$

Mathematics Formulae

Displacement along x axis at any instant t is	Displacement along y axis at any instant t is
$x = u_x t + \dfrac{1}{2} a_x t^2$	$y = u_y t + \dfrac{1}{2} a_y t^2$
$x = u_x t + 0$	$y = 0 + \dfrac{1}{2} a_y t^2$
$x = ut$	$y = \dfrac{1}{2} g t^2$

Note: The horizontal component of velocity does not change throughout the projectile motion.

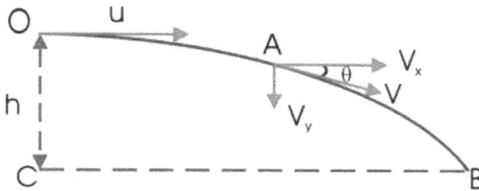

Total Velocity at any instant of time t

At instant of time t, $v_x = u$ and $v_y = gt$, hence

$$v = (v_x^2 + v_y^2)^{1/2} = [u^2 + (gt)^2]^{1/2}$$

Angular Projection

Let a body of mass m be projected into the air with velocity u in a direction making an angle θ with the horizontal. Let origin O of the coordinate axes be the point of projection.

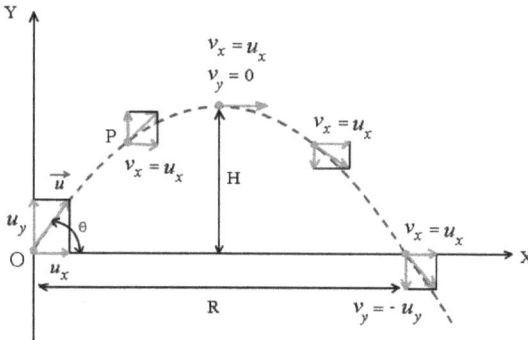

Let P(x, y) be the position of the body after time t. During the projectile motion, the only force which acts on the body is its weight which acts downwards.

(i) The equation of motion along x axis is

$$m\frac{d^2x}{dt^2} = 0 \text{ or } \frac{d^2x}{dt^2} = 0$$

Integrating both sides, we get $\frac{dx}{dt}$ = c where c is the constant of integration

Initially at the origin, time = 0 and $u_x = u \cos \theta$

Therefore, $v_x = \frac{dx}{dt}$ $u \cos \theta$

Integrating again and applying initial conditions we get, $x = u \cos \theta . t$

(ii) The equation of motion along y axis is

$$m\frac{d^2y}{dt^2} = -mg \text{ Or } \frac{d^2y}{dt^2} = -g$$

Integrating both sides, we get $\frac{dy}{dt} = -gt + k$, where k is the constant of integration

Initially at the origin, time = 0 and $u_y = u \sin \theta$

Therefore $\frac{dy}{dt} = u \sin \theta - gt$

Integrating again and applying initial conditions, we get

$$y = u \sin \theta . t - \frac{1}{2} gt^2$$

Along x axis	Along y axis
Component of initial velocity along x axis is $u_x = u \cos \theta$	Component of initial velocity along y axis is $u_y = u \sin \theta$
Acceleration along x axis is $a_x = 0$	Acceleration along y axis is $a_y = -g$
Component of velocity along x axis at any instant t is $v_x = u \cos \theta$	Component of velocity along y axis at any instant t is $v_y = u \sin \theta - gt$
Displacement along x axis at any instant t is $x = u \cos \theta . t$	Displacement along y axis at any instant t is $y = u\sin\theta . t - \frac{1}{2} gt^2$

Mathematics Formulae

Important Terms Associated with Projectile

The objects that are projected from a horizontal surface and land on the same horizontal surface have a vertically symmetrical path.

Path of a Projectile

The path of a projectile is called its *trajectory*. The path of a projectile is a parabola.

Equation of trajectory

$$y = x \tan\theta - \frac{1}{2} g \, u^2 \sec^2 \theta . \, x^2$$

Time of Flight

The time it takes for an object to be projected and landing back on the surface is known as time of flight. It depends on the initial velocity of the object and the angle of projection. $T = \frac{2u \sin\theta}{g}$

Range

The horizontal displacement of the projectile is known as the range of the projectile. It depends on the initial velocity of the object and the angle of projection.

$$R = \frac{u^2 \sin 2\theta}{g}$$

Maximum Range

The range will be maximum when $\sin 2\theta = 1$ or $\theta = 45°$

$$R = \frac{u^2}{g}$$

Maximum Height

The maximum height is attained by the projectile when the projectile reaches zero vertical velocity. At this point gravity accelerates the body downwards.

$$H = \frac{u^2 \sin^2 \theta}{2g}$$

Appendix

MATHEMATICAL CONSTANTS

The square root of 2 is known as Pythagoras's constant.

Continued Fraction

$$\sqrt{2} = 1 + \cfrac{1}{2 + \cfrac{1}{2 + \cfrac{1}{2 + \cfrac{1}{2 + \cfrac{1}{2 + \ddots}}}}}$$

Geometrical Representation

is equal to the length of the hypotenuse of a right angled triangle with sides one.

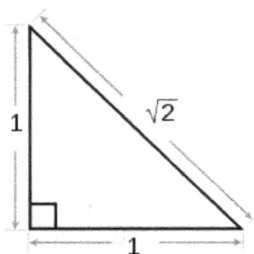

The square root of 3 is known as Theodorus's constant. Theodorus proved that the square roots of the numbers from 3 to 17 (excluding 4, 9 and 16) are irrational.

Continued Fraction
The continued fraction of 3 is given by:

$$\sqrt{3} = 1 + \cfrac{1}{1 + \cfrac{1}{2 + \cfrac{1}{1 + \cfrac{1}{2 + \cfrac{1}{1 + \cdots}}}}}$$

Geometrical Representation

Geometrically $\sqrt{3}$ represents the diagonal of a unit cube.

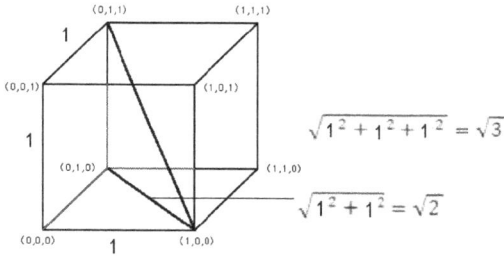

$$\sqrt{1^2 + 1^2 + 1^2} = \sqrt{3}$$

$$\sqrt{1^2 + 1^2} = \sqrt{2}$$

Archimedes' Constant π

The ratio between the circumference and the diameter of a circle is known as pi. It is an irrational as well as a transcendental (it is not the solution of any polynomial equation with rational coefficients) number.

$$\pi = 3.14159265358979323846$$

Continued Fraction

The continued fraction of π is given by:

$$\pi = \cfrac{4}{1 + \cfrac{1^2}{2 + \cfrac{3^2}{2 + \cfrac{5^2}{2 + \cfrac{7^2}{2 + \cfrac{9^2}{2 + \cdots}}}}}} = 3 + \cfrac{1^2}{6 + \cfrac{3^2}{6 + \cfrac{5^2}{6 + \cfrac{7^2}{6 + \cfrac{9^2}{6 + \cdots}}}}} = \cfrac{4}{1 + \cfrac{1^2}{3 + \cfrac{2^2}{5 + \cfrac{3^2}{7 + \cfrac{4^2}{9 + \cdots}}}}}$$

Infinite Series

The infinite series of π is given by

$$\pi = \frac{4}{1} - \frac{4}{3} + \frac{4}{5} - \frac{4}{7} + \frac{4}{9} - \frac{4}{11} + \frac{4}{13} - \cdots$$

$$\pi = 3 + \frac{4}{2 \times 3 \times 4} - \frac{4}{4 \times 5 \times 6} + \frac{4}{6 \times 7 \times 8} - \frac{4}{8 \times 9 \times 10} + \cdots$$

Euler's Number *e*

The exponential growth constant *e* is defined as

$$e = \lim_{n \to \infty} \left(1 + \frac{1}{n}\right)^2$$

It is an irrational number.

$e = 2.71828182845904523536028747135 2$

Continued Fraction

$$e = 2 + \cfrac{1}{1 + \cfrac{1}{2 + \cfrac{1}{1 + \cfrac{1}{1 + \cfrac{1}{4 + \cfrac{1}{1 + \cfrac{1}{1 + \cdots}}}}}}} = 1 + \cfrac{1}{0 + \cfrac{1}{1 + \cfrac{1}{1 + \cfrac{1}{2 + \cfrac{1}{1 + \cfrac{1}{1 + \cfrac{1}{4 + \cfrac{1}{1 + \cfrac{1}{1 + \cdots}}}}}}}}}$$

Infinite Series

$$e = \frac{1}{1!} + \frac{1}{2!} + \frac{1}{3!} + \frac{1}{4!} + \ldots$$

Geometric Representation

The value of $(1 + 1/n)^n$ approaches *e* as *n* gets bigger and bigger.

n	$(1 + 1/n)^n$
1	2.00000
2	2.25000
5	2.48832
10	2.59374
100	2.70481
1,000	2.71692
10,000	2.71815
100,000	2.71827

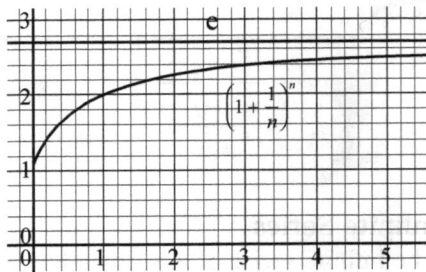

Imaginary Number *i*

A real number multiplied by the imaginary unit *i* gives an imaginary number. Imaginary numbers (except 0) produce negative real numbers when squared (0 is both real and imaginary).

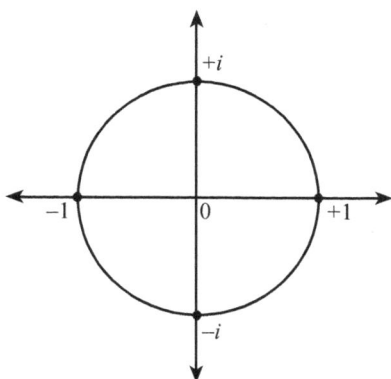

Property of Imaginary Number i

$$i^2 = -1$$
$$i^3 = -i = \frac{1}{i}$$
$$i^4 = 1$$
$$i^{-3} = i$$

Link Between Imaginary Number and Sine, Cosine

The imaginary number 'i' provides a link between 'e' and the trigonometric functions sin and cos, thus uniting two branches of mathematics. For example, De Moivre's theorem gives

$$(\cos x + i \sin x)^n = \cos nx + i \sin nx$$

which appears more naturally as

$$(e^{ix})^n = e^{inx}$$

Golden Ratio ϕ

Two quantities are in the golden ratio if their ratio is the same as the ratio of their sum to the larger of the two quantities.

Algebraic Representation

Algebraically, for two quantities a and b with $a > b$,

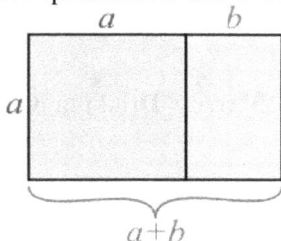

$$\phi = \frac{a+b}{a} = \frac{a}{b}$$

Arithmetic Representation

Arithmetically (phi) is given as:

$$= \frac{1+\sqrt{5}}{2}$$

Continued Fraction

The continued fraction of is given by:

$$= 1 + \cfrac{1}{1 + \cfrac{1}{1 + \cfrac{1}{1 + \ldots}}}$$

The number 1 followed by a googol of zeroes is known as googolplex.

Fun fact: *'Google'* *the most used search engine on the internet has* **Googol***. It was*

CONVERSION OF UNITS

A mnemonic is a pattern of letters, ideas, word, sentence, poem etc. which helps us in remembering something.

Metric System

measures in order.

King Henry Danced Merrily Drinking Chocolate Milk

Imperial System

1 Foot(ft)	=	12 Inches (in)
1 Mile(mi)	=	5280 Feet (ft)
1 Mile (mi)	=	1760 Yard (yd)
1 Yard (yd)	=	3 Feet (ft)

Conversion from metric system to imperial system

1 Kilometre (km)	=	0.6214 Mile (mi)
1 Metre (m)	=	1.0936 Yard (yd)
1 Centimetre (cm)	=	0.3937 Inch (in)
1 Millimetre (mm)	=	0.03937 Inch (in)

Conversion from imperial system to metric system

1 Inches (in)	=	2.54 Centimetre (cm)
1 Foot (ft)	=	0.3048 Metre (m)
1 Mile(mi)	=	1.6093 Kilometre (km)
1 Yard (yd)	=	0.9144 Metre (m)

Area Measure

Metric System

1 Sq.km(km^2)	=	100 Hectare (ha)
1 Hectare (ha)	=	10,000 Sq.m (m^2)
1 Sq.m (m^2)	=	10,000 Sq.cm (cm^2)
1 Sq.cm (cm^2)	=	100 Sq.mm (mm^2)

Imperial System

1 Sq.ft (ft^2)	=	144 Sq.in (in^2)
1 Sq.yd (yd^2)	=	9 Sq.ft (ft^2)
1 Acre	=	4840 Sq.yd (yd^2)
1 Sq.mi(mile ^{2})	=	640 Acres

Conversion from metric system to imperial system

1 Sq.km (km^2)	=	0.3861 Sq.mile (mile^2)
1 Hectare (ha)	=	2.4711 Acres
1 Sq.m (m^2)	=	1.1960 Sq.yd (yd^2)
1 Sq.cm (cm^2)	=	0.1550 Sq.in (in^2)

Conversion from imperial system to metric system

1 Sq.in (in^2)	=	6.4516 Sq.cm(cm^2)
1 Sq.ft (ft^2)	=	0.0929 Sq.m (m^2)
1 Sq.yd (yd^2)	=	0.8361 Sq.m(m^2)
1 Acre	=	4046.86 Sq.m (m^2)
1 Sq.mi(mile ^{2})	=	2.589 Sq.km (km^2)

Mass Measure

The first letters of the mnemonic indicates the first letters of the weight measures in order.

King	**Henry**	**Danced**	**Grandly**	**Drinking**	**Chocolate**	**Milk**
Kilo	Hecto	Deca	Gram	Deci	Centi	Milli

Metric System

1 Tonne	=	1000 Kilogram (kg)
1 Kilogram (kg)	=	1000 Gram (g)
1 Gram (g)	=	1000 Milligram (mg)

Imperial System

1 Stone	=	14 Pound (lb)
1 Pound (lb)	=	16 Ounce (oz)
1 Ounce (oz)	=	437.5 Grain

Conversion from metric system to imperial system

1 Tonne	=	0.9842 Long ton
1 Tonne	=	1.1023 Short ton
1 Kilogram (kg)	=	2.2046 Pound (lb)
1 Gram (g)	=	0.0353 Ounce (oz)
1 Milligram (mg)	=	0.0154 Grain

Conversion from imperial system to metric system

1 Long ton	=	1.0160 Tonne
1 Short ton	=	0.9072 Tonne
1 Stone	=	6.3503 Kilogram (kg)
1 Pound (lb)	=	0.4536 Kilogram (kg)
1 Ounce (oz)	=	28.349 Gram (g)

Volume Measure

The first letters of the mnemonic indicates the first letters of the weight measures in order.

King	**Henry**	**Danced**	**Lazily**	**Drinking**	**Chocolate**	**Milk**
Kilo	Hecto	Deca	Litre	Deci	Centi	Milli

Metric System

1 Litre(l)	=	1 Cu.dm (dm^3)
1 Cu.m (m^3)	=	1000 Cu.dm(dm^3)
1 Cu.dm(dm^3)	=	1000 Cu.cm(cm^3)

Imperial System

1 Gallon (gal)	=	4 Quarts (qt) or 16 Cups (c)
1 Quart (qt)	=	2 Pints (pt) or 4 Cups(c)

1 Pint (pt)	=	2 Cups (c) or 16 Fluid ounce (oz)
1 Cup (c)	=	8 Fluid ounce (oz)

Conversion from metric system to imperial system

1 Litre(l)	=	1.7598 Pint (pt)
1 Cu.m (m^3)	=	1.30795 Cu.yd (yd^3)
1 Cu.dm(dm^3)	=	0.0353 Cu.ft (ft^3)
1 Cu.cm (cm^3)	=	0.0610 Cu.in (in^3)

Conversion from imperial system to metric system

1 Gallon (gal)	=	3.7854 Litre (l)
1 Pint (pt)	=	0.4732 Litre (l)
1 Fluid ounce (oz)	=	29.5735 Millilitre (ml)
1 Cu.ft (ft^3)	=	0.02832 Cu.m (m^3)
1 Cu.in(in^3)	=	16.387 Cu.cm (cm^3)

Measure of Time

1 Century	=	100 Years (yrs)
1 Decade	=	10 Years (yr)
1 Years (yr)	=	12 Months
1 Month	=	30 or 31 Days (except February)
February month	=	28 Days (non leap year)
February month	=	29 Days (leap year)
1 Year (yr)	=	52 Weeks
1 Week	=	7 Days
1 Years (yr)	=	365 Days (non leap year)
1 Years (yr)	=	366 Days (leap year)
1 Day	=	24 Hours (hr)
1 Hour (hr)	=	60 Minutes (min)
1 Minute (min)	=	60 Seconds (sec)
Midnight	=	0000 Hour
Noon	=	1200 Hour

A leap year occurs once in four years.

Measure of Temperature

The international standard unit of temperature is Kelvin (K). Other commonly used units are Celsius (C) and Fahrenheit (F).

Boiling point of water = 100 °C = 212 °F = 373.15 K

Freezing point of water = 0 °C = 32 °F = 273.15 K

LOGARITHM AND ANTILOGARITHM TABLES

x	0.00	0.01	0.02	0.03	0.04	0.05	0.06	0.07	0.08	0.09
1.0	.0000	.0043	.0086	.0128	.0170	.0212	.0253	.0294	.0334	.0374
1.1	.0414	.0453	.0492	.0531	.0569	.0607	.0645	.0682	.0719	.0755
1.2	.0792	.0828	.0864	.0899	.0934	.0969	.1004	.1038	.1072	.1106
1.3	.1139	.1173	.1206	.1239	.1271	.1303	.1335	.1367	.1399	.1430
1.4	.1461	.1492	.1523	.1553	.1584	.1614	.1644	.1673	.1703	.1732
1.5	.1761	.1790	.1818	.1847	.1875	.1903	.1931	.1959	.1987	.2014
1.6	.2041	.2068	.2095	.2122	.2148	.2175	.2201	.2227	.2253	.2279
1.7	.2304	.2330	.2355	.2380	.2405	.2430	.2455	.2480	.2504	.2529
1.8	.2553	.2577	.2601	.2625	.2648	.2672	.2695	.2718	.2742	.2765
1.9	.2788	.2810	.2833	.2856	.2878	.2900	.2923	.2945	.2967	.2989
2.0	.3010	.3032	.3054	.3075	.3096	.3118	.3139	.3160	.3181	.3201
2.1	.3222	.3243	.3263	.3284	.3304	.3324	.3345	.3365	.3385	.3404
2.2	.3424	.3444	.3464	.3483	.3502	.3522	.3541	.3560	.3579	.3598
2.3	.3617	.3636	.3655	.3674	.3692	.3711	.3729	.3747	.3766	.3784
2.4	.3802	.3820	.3838	.3856	.3874	.3892	.3909	.3927	.3945	.3962
2.5	.3979	.3997	.4014	.4031	.4048	.4065	.4082	.4099	.4116	.4133
2.6	.4150	.4166	.4183	.4200	.4216	.4232	.4249	.4265	.4281	.4298
2.7	.4314	.4330	.4346	.4362	.4378	.4393	.4409	.4425	.4440	.4456
2.8	.4472	.4487	.4502	.4518	.4533	.4548	.4564	.4579	.4594	.4609
2.9	.4624	.4639	.4654	.4669	.4683	.4698	.4713	.4728	.4742	.4757
3.0	.4771	.4786	.4800	.4814	.4829	.4843	.4857	.4871	.4886	.4900
3.1	.4914	.4928	.4942	.4955	.4969	.4983	.4997	.5011	.5024	.5038
3.2	.5051	.5065	.5079	.5092	.5105	.5119	.5132	.5145	.5159	.5172
3.3	.5185	.5198	.5211	.5224	.5237	.5250	.5263	.5276	.5289	.5302
3.4	.5315	.5328	.5340	.5353	.5366	.5378	.5391	.5403	.5416	.5428
3.5	.5441	.5453	.5465	.5478	.5490	.5502	.5514	.5527	.5539	.5551
3.6	.5563	.5575	.5587	.5599	.5611	.5623	.5635	.5647	.5658	.5670
3.7	.5682	.5694	.5705	.5717	.5729	.5740	.5752	.5763	.5775	.5786
3.8	.5798	.5809	.5821	.5832	.5843	.5855	.5866	.5877	.5888	.5899
3.9	.5911	.5922	.5933	.5944	.5955	.5966	.5977	.5988	.5999	.6010
4.0	.6021	.6031	.6042	.6053	.6064	.6075	.6085	.6096	.6107	.6117
4.1	.6128	.6138	.6149	.6160	.6170	.6180	.6191	.6201	.6212	.6222
4.2	.6232	.6243	.6253	.6263	.6274	.6284	.6294	.6304	.6314	.6325
4.3	.6335	.6345	.6355	.6365	.6375	.6385	.6395	.6405	.6415	.6425
4.4	.6435	.6444	.6454	.6464	.6474	.6484	.6493	.6503	.6513	.6522
4.5	.6532	.6542	.6551	.6561	.6571	.6580	.6590	.6599	.6609	.6618
4.6	.6628	.6637	.6646	.6656	.6665	.6675	.6684	.6693	.6702	.6712
4.7	.6721	.6730	.6739	.6749	.6758	.6767	.6776	.6785	.6794	.6803
4.8	.6812	.6821	.6830	.6839	.6848	.6857	.6866	.6875	.6884	.6893
4.9	.6902	.6911	.6920	.6928	.6937	.6946	.6955	.6964	.6972	.6981
5.0	.6990	.6998	.7007	.7016	.7024	.7033	.7042	.7050	.7059	.7067
5.1	.7076	.7084	.7093	.7101	.7110	.7118	.7126	.7135	.7143	.7152
5.2	.7160	.7168	.7177	.7185	.7193	.7202	.7210	.7218	.7226	.7235
5.3	.7243	.7251	.7259	.7267	.7275	.7284	.7292	.7300	.7308	.7316
5.4	.7324	.7332	.7340	.7348	.7356	.7364	.7372	.7380	.7388	.7396

x	0.00	0.01	0.02	0.03	0.04	0.05	0.06	0.07	0.08	0.09
5.5	.7404	.7412	.7419	.7427	.7435	.7443	.7451	.7459	.7466	.7474
5.6	.7482	.7490	.7497	.7505	.7513	.7520	.7528	.7536	.7543	.7551
5.7	.7559	.7566	.7574	.7582	.7589	.7597	.7604	.7612	.7619	.7627
5.8	.7634	.7642	.7649	.7657	.7664	.7672	.7679	.7686	.7694	.7701
5.9	.7709	.7716	.7723	.7731	.7738	.7745	.7752	.7760	.7767	.7774
6.0	.7782	.7789	.7796	.7803	.7810	.7818	.7825	.7832	.7839	.7846
6.1	.7853	.7860	.7868	.7875	.7882	.7889	.7896	.7903	.7910	.7917
6.2	.7924	.7931	.7938	.7945	.7952	.7959	.7966	.7973	.7980	.7987
6.3	.7993	.8000	.8007	.8014	.8021	.8028	.8035	.8041	.8048	.8055
6.4	.8062	.8069	.8075	.8082	.8089	.8096	.8102	.8109	.8116	.8122
6.5	.8129	.8136	.8142	.8149	.8156	.8162	.8169	.8176	.8182	.8189
6.6	.8195	.8202	.8209	.8215	.8222	.8228	.8235	.8241	.8248	.8254
6.7	.8261	.8267	.8274	.8280	.8287	.8293	.8299	.8306	.8312	.8319
6.8	.8325	.8331	.8338	.8344	.8351	.8357	.8363	.8370	.8376	.8382
6.9	.8388	.8395	.8401	.8407	.8414	.8420	.8426	.8432	.8439	.8445
7.0	.8451	.8457	.8463	.8470	.8476	.8482	.8488	.8494	.8500	.8506
7.1	.8513	.8519	.8525	.8531	.8537	.8543	.8549	.8555	.8561	.8567
7.2	.8573	.8579	.8585	.8591	.8597	.8603	.8609	.8615	.8621	.8627
7.3	.8633	.8639	.8645	.8651	.8657	.8663	.8669	.8675	.8681	.8686
7.4	.8692	.8698	.8704	.8710	.8716	.8722	.8727	.8733	.8739	.8745
7.5	.8751	.8756	.8762	.8768	.8774	.8779	.8785	.8791	.8797	.8802
7.6	.8808	.8814	.8820	.8825	.8831	.8837	.8842	.8848	.8854	.8859
7.7	.8865	.8871	.8876	.8882	.8887	.8893	.8899	.8904	.8910	.8915
7.8	.8921	.8927	.8932	.8938	.8943	.8949	.8954	.8960	.8965	.8971
7.9	.8976	.8982	.8987	.8993	.8998	.9004	.9009	.9015	.9020	.9025
8.0	.9031	.9036	.9042	.9047	.9053	.9058	.9063	.9069	.9074	.9079
8.1	.9085	.9090	.9096	.9101	.9106	.9112	.9117	.9122	.9128	.9133
8.2	.9138	.9143	.9149	.9154	.9159	.9165	.9170	.9175	.9180	.9186
8.3	.9191	.9196	.9201	.9206	.9212	.9217	.9222	.9227	.9232	.9238
8.4	.9243	.9248	.9253	.9258	.9263	.9269	.9274	.9279	.9284	.9289
8.5	.9294	.9299	.9304	.9309	.9315	.9320	.9325	.9330	.9335	.9340
8.6	.9345	.9350	.9355	.9360	.9365	.9370	.9375	.9380	.9385	.9390
8.7	.9395	.9400	.9405	.9410	.9415	.9420	.9425	.9430	.9435	.9440
8.8	.9445	.9450	.9455	.9460	.9465	.9469	.9474	.9479	.9484	.9489
8.9	.9494	.9499	.9504	.9509	.9513	.9518	.9523	.9528	.9533	.9538
9.0	.9542	.9547	.9552	.9557	.9562	.9566	.9571	.9576	.9581	.9586
9.1	.9590	.9595	.9600	.9605	.9609	.9614	.9619	.9624	.9628	.9633
9.2	.9638	.9643	.9647	.9652	.9657	.9661	.9666	.9671	.9675	.9680
9.3	.9685	.9689	.9694	.9699	.9703	.9708	.9713	.9717	.9722	.9727
9.4	.9731	.9736	.9741	.9745	.9750	.9754	.9759	.9763	.9768	.9773
9.5	.9777	.9782	.9786	.9791	.9795	.9800	.9805	.9809	.9814	.9818
9.6	.9823	.9827	.9832	.9836	.9841	.9845	.9850	.9854	.9859	.9863
9.7	.9868	.9872	.9877	.9881	.9886	.9890	.9894	.9899	.9903	.9908
9.8	.9912	.9917	.9921	.9926	.9930	.9934	.9939	.9943	.9948	.9952
9.9	.9956	.9961	.9965	.9969	.9974	.9978	.9983	.9987	.9991	.9996

	0	1	2	3	4	5	6	7	8	9
·00	1000	1002	1005	1007	1009	1012	1014	1016	1019	1021
·01	1023	1026	1028	1030	1033	1035	1038	1040	1042	1045
·02	1047	1050	1052	1054	1057	1059	1062	1064	1067	1069
·03	1072	1074	1076	1079	1081	1084	1086	1089	1091	1094
·04	1096	1099	1102	1104	1107	1109	1112	1114	1117	1119
·05	1122	1125	1127	1130	1132	1135	1138	1140	1143	1146
·06	1148	1151	1153	1156	1159	1161	1164	1167	1169	1172
·07	1175	1178	1180	1183	1186	1189	1191	1194	1197	1199
·08	1202	1205	1208	1211	1213	1216	1219	1222	1225	1227
·09	1230	1233	1236	1239	1242	1245	1247	1250	1253	1256
·10	1259	1262	1265	1268	1271	1274	1276	1279	1282	1285
·11	1288	1291	1294	1297	1300	1303	1306	1309	1312	1315
·12	1318	1321	1324	1327	1330	1334	1337	1340	1343	1346
·13	1349	1352	1355	1358	1361	1365	1368	1371	1374	1377
·14	1380	1384	1387	1390	1393	1396	1400	1403	1406	1409
·15	1413	1416	1419	1422	1426	1429	1432	1435	1439	1442
·16	1445	1449	1452	1455	1459	1462	1466	1469	1472	1476
·17	1479	1483	1486	1489	1493	1496	1500	1503	1507	1510
·18	1514	1517	1521	1524	1528	1531	1535	1538	1542	1545
·19	1549	1552	1556	1560	1563	1567	1570	1574	1578	1581
·20	1585	1589	1592	1596	1600	1603	1607	1611	1614	1618
·21	1622	1626	1629	1633	1637	1641	1644	1648	1652	1656
·22	1660	1663	1667	1671	1675	1679	1683	1687	1690	1694
·23	1698	1702	1706	1710	1714	1718	1722	1726	1730	1734
·24	1738	1742	1746	1750	1754	1758	1762	1766	1770	1774
·25	1778	1782	1786	1791	1795	1799	1803	1807	1811	1816
·26	1820	1824	1828	1832	1837	1841	1845	1849	1854	1858
·27	1862	1866	1871	1875	1879	1884	1888	1892	1897	1901
·28	1905	1910	1914	1919	1923	1928	1932	1936	1941	1945
·29	1950	1954	1959	1963	1968	1972	1977	1982	1986	1991
·30	1995	2000	2004	2009	2014	2018	2023	2028	2032	2037
·31	2042	2046	2051	2056	2061	2065	2070	2075	2080	2084
·32	2089	2094	2099	2104	2109	2113	2118	2123	2128	2133
·33	2138	2143	2148	2153	2158	2163	2168	2173	2178	2183
·34	2188	2193	2198	2203	2208	2213	2218	2223	2228	2234
·35	2239	2244	2249	2254	2259	2265	2270	2275	2280	2286
·36	2291	2296	2301	2307	2312	2317	2323	2328	2333	2339
·37	2344	2350	2355	2360	2366	2371	2377	2382	2388	2393
·38	2399	2404	2410	2415	2421	2427	2432	2438	2443	2449
·39	2455	2460	2466	2472	2477	2483	2489	2495	2500	2506
·40	2512	2518	2523	2529	2535	2541	2547	2553	2559	2564
·41	2570	2576	2582	2588	2594	2600	2606	2612	2618	2624
·42	2630	2636	2642	2649	2655	2661	2667	2673	2679	2685
·43	2692	2698	2704	2710	2716	2723	2729	2735	2742	2748
·44	2754	2761	2767	2773	2780	2786	2793	2799	2805	2812
·45	2818	2825	2831	2838	2844	2851	2858	2864	2871	2877
·46	2884	2891	2897	2904	2911	2917	2924	2931	2938	2944
·47	2951	2958	2965	2972	2970	2985	2992	2999	3006	3013
·48	3020	3027	3034	3041	3048	3055	3062	3069	3076	3083
·49	3090	3097	3105	3112	3119	3126	3133	3141	3148	3155

	0	1	2	3	4	5	6	7	8	9
·50	3162	3170	3177	3184	3192	3199	3206	3214	3221	3228
·51	3236	3243	3251	3258	3266	3273	3281	3289	3296	3304
·52	3311	3319	3327	3334	3342	3350	3357	3365	3373	3381
·53	3388	3396	3404	3412	3420	3428	3436	3443	3451	3459
·54	3467	3475	3483	3491	3499	3508	3516	3524	3532	3540
·55	3548	3556	3565	3573	3581	3589	3597	3606	3614	3622
·56	3631	3639	3648	3656	3664	3673	3681	3690	3698	3707
·57	3715	3724	3733	3741	3750	3758	3767	3776	3784	3793
·58	3802	3811	3819	3828	3837	3846	3855	3864	3873	3882
·59	3890	3899	3908	3917	3926	3936	3945	3954	3963	3972
·60	3981	3990	3999	4009	4018	4027	4036	4046	4055	4064
·61	4074	4083	4093	4102	4111	4121	4130	4140	4150	4159
·62	4169	4178	4188	4198	4207	4217	4227	4236	4246	4256
·63	4266	4276	4285	4295	4305	4315	4325	4335	4345	4355
·64	4365	4375	4385	4395	4406	4416	4426	4436	4446	4457
·65	4467	4477	4487	4498	4508	4519	4529	4539	4550	4560
·66	4571	4581	4592	4603	4613	4624	4634	4645	4656	4667
·67	4677	4688	4699	4710	4721	4732	4742	4753	4764	4775
·68	4786	4797	4808	4819	4831	4842	4853	4864	4875	4887
·69	4898	4909	4920	4932	4943	4955	4966	4977	4989	5000
·70	5012	5023	5035	5047	5058	5070	5082	5093	5105	5117
·71	5129	5140	5152	5164	5176	5188	5200	5212	5224	5236
·72	5248	5260	5272	5284	5297	5309	5321	5333	5346	5358
·73	5370	5383	5395	5408	5420	5433	5445	5458	5470	5483
·74	5495	5508	5521	5534	5546	5559	5572	5585	5598	5610
·75	5623	5636	5649	5662	5675	5689	5702	5715	5728	5741
·76	5754	5768	5781	5794	5808	5821	5834	5848	5861	5875
·77	5888	5902	5916	5929	5943	5957	5970	5984	5998	6012
·78	6026	6039	6053	6067	6081	6095	6109	6124	6138	6152
·79	6166	6180	6194	6209	6223	6237	6252	6266	6281	6295
·80	6310	6324	6339	6353	6368	6383	6397	6412	6427	6442
·81	6457	6471	6486	6501	6516	6531	6546	6561	6577	6592
·82	6607	6622	6637	6653	6668	6683	6699	6714	6730	6745
·83	6761	6776	6792	6808	6823	6839	6855	6871	6887	6902
·84	6918	6934	6950	6966	6982	6998	7015	7031	7047	7063
·85	7079	7096	7112	7129	7145	7161	7178	7194	7211	7228
·86	7244	7261	7278	7295	7311	7328	7345	7362	7379	7396
·87	7413	7430	7447	7464	7482	7499	7516	7534	7551	7568
·88	7586	7603	7621	7638	7656	7674	7691	7709	7727	7745
·89	7762	7780	7798	7816	7834	7852	7870	7889	7907	7925
·90	7943	7962	7980	7998	8017	8035	8054	8072	8091	8110
·91	8128	8147	8166	8185	8204	8222	8241	8260	8279	8299
·92	8318	8337	8356	8375	8395	8414	8433	8453	8472	8492
·93	8511	8531	8551	8570	8590	8610	8630	8650	8670	8690
·94	8710	8730	8750	8770	8790	8810	8831	8851	8872	8892
·95	8913	8933	8954	8974	8995	9016	9036	9057	9078	9099
·96	9120	9141	9162	9183	9204	9226	9247	9268	9290	9311
·97	9333	9354	9376	9397	9419	9441	9462	9484	9506	9528
·98	9550	9572	9594	9616	9638	9661	9683	9705	9727	9750
·99	9772	9795	9817	9840	9863	9886	9908	9931	9954	9977

TRIGONOMETRIC TABLES

x deg	x rad	sin(x)	cos(x)	tan(x)	cot(x)	csc(x)	sec(x)
0	0	0.0000	1.0000	0.0000			1.0000
1	0.0175	0.0175	0.9998	0.0175	57.2900	57.2987	1.0002
2	0.0349	0.0349	0.9994	0.0349	28.6363	28.6537	1.0006
3	0.0524	0.0523	0.9986	0.0524	19.0811	19.1073	1.0014
4	0.0698	0.0698	0.9976	0.0699	14.3007	14.3356	1.0024
5	0.0873	0.0872	0.9962	0.0875	11.4301	11.4737	1.0038
6	0.1047	0.1045	0.9945	0.1051	9.5144	9.5668	1.0055
7	0.1222	0.1219	0.9925	0.1228	8.1443	8.2055	1.0075
8	0.1396	0.1392	0.9903	0.1405	7.1154	7.1853	1.0098
9	0.1571	0.1564	0.9877	0.1584	6.3138	6.3925	1.0125
10	0.1745	0.1736	0.9848	0.1763	5.6713	5.7588	1.0154
11	0.192	0.1908	0.9816	0.1944	5.1446	5.2408	1.0187
12	0.2094	0.2079	0.9781	0.2126	4.7046	4.8097	1.0223
13	0.2269	0.2250	0.9744	0.2309	4.3315	4.4454	1.0263
14	0.2443	0.2419	0.9703	0.2493	4.0108	4.1336	1.0306
15	0.2618	0.2588	0.9659	0.2679	3.7321	3.8637	1.0353
16	0.2793	0.2756	0.9613	0.2867	3.4874	3.6280	1.0403
17	0.2967	0.2924	0.9563	0.3057	3.2709	3.4203	1.0457
18	0.3142	0.3090	0.9511	0.3249	3.0777	3.2361	1.0515
19	0.3316	0.3256	0.9455	0.3443	2.9042	3.0716	1.0576
20	0.3491	0.3420	0.9397	0.3640	2.7475	2.9238	1.0642
21	0.3665	0.3584	0.9336	0.3839	2.6051	2.7904	1.0711
22	0.384	0.3746	0.9272	0.4040	2.4751	2.6695	1.0785
23	0.4014	0.3907	0.9205	0.4245	2.3559	2.5593	1.0864
24	0.4189	0.4067	0.9135	0.4452	2.2460	2.4586	1.0946
25	0.4363	0.4226	0.9063	0.4663	2.1445	2.3662	1.1034
26	0.4538	0.4384	0.8988	0.4877	2.0503	2.2812	1.1126
27	0.4712	0.4540	0.8910	0.5095	1.9626	2.2027	1.1223
28	0.4887	0.4695	0.8829	0.5317	1.8807	2.1301	1.1326
29	0.5061	0.4848	0.8746	0.5543	1.8040	2.0627	1.1434
30	0.5236	0.5000	0.8660	0.5774	1.7321	2.0000	1.1547
31	0.5411	0.5150	0.8572	0.6009	1.6643	1.9416	1.1666
32	0.5585	0.5299	0.8480	0.6249	1.6003	1.8871	1.1792
33	0.576	0.5446	0.8387	0.6494	1.5399	1.8361	1.1924
34	0.5934	0.5592	0.8290	0.6745	1.4826	1.7883	1.2062
35	0.6109	0.5736	0.8192	0.7002	1.4281	1.7434	1.2208
36	0.6283	0.5878	0.8090	0.7265	1.3764	1.7013	1.2361
37	0.6458	0.6018	0.7986	0.7536	1.3270	1.6616	1.2521
38	0.6632	0.6157	0.7880	0.7813	1.2799	1.6243	1.2690
39	0.6807	0.6293	0.7771	0.8098	1.2349	1.5890	1.2868
40	0.6981	0.6428	0.7660	0.8391	1.1918	1.5557	1.3054
41	0.7156	0.6561	0.7547	0.8693	1.1504	1.5243	1.3250
42	0.733	0.6691	0.7431	0.9004	1.1106	1.4945	1.3456
43	0.7505	0.6820	0.7314	0.9325	1.0724	1.4663	1.3673
44	0.7679	0.6947	0.7193	0.9657	1.0355	1.4396	1.3902
45	0.7854	0.7071	0.7071	1.0000	1.0000	1.4142	1.4142

x		sin(x)	cos(x)	tan(x)	cot(x)	csc(x)	sec(x)
deg	rad						
46	0.8029	0.7193	0.6947	1.0355	0.9657	1.3902	1.4396
47	0.8203	0.7314	0.6820	1.0724	0.9325	1.3673	1.4663
48	0.8378	0.7431	0.6691	1.1106	0.9004	1.3456	1.4945
49	0.8552	0.7547	0.6561	1.1504	0.8693	1.3250	1.5243
50	0.8727	0.7660	0.6428	1.1918	0.8391	1.3054	1.5557
51	0.8901	0.7771	0.6293	1.2349	0.8098	1.2868	1.5890
52	0.9076	0.7880	0.6157	1.2799	0.7813	1.2690	1.6243
53	0.925	0.7986	0.6018	1.3270	0.7536	1.2521	1.6616
54	0.9425	0.8090	0.5878	1.3764	0.7265	1.2361	1.7013
55	0.9599	0.8192	0.5736	1.4281	0.7002	1.2208	1.7434
56	0.9774	0.8290	0.5592	1.4826	0.6745	1.2062	1.7883
57	0.9948	0.8387	0.5446	1.5399	0.6494	1.1924	1.8361
58	1.0123	0.8480	0.5299	1.6003	0.6249	1.1792	1.8871
59	1.0297	0.8572	0.5150	1.6643	0.6009	1.1666	1.9416
60	1.0472	0.8660	0.5000	1.7321	0.5774	1.1547	2.0000
61	1.0647	0.8746	0.4848	1.8040	0.5543	1.1434	2.0627
62	1.0821	0.8829	0.4695	1.8807	0.5317	1.1326	2.1301
63	1.0996	0.8910	0.4540	1.9626	0.5095	1.1223	2.2027
64	1.117	0.8988	0.4384	2.0503	0.4877	1.1126	2.2812
65	1.1345	0.9063	0.4226	2.1445	0.4663	1.1034	2.3662
66	1.1519	0.9135	0.4067	2.2460	0.4452	1.0946	2.4586
67	1.1694	0.9205	0.3907	2.3559	0.4245	1.0864	2.5593
68	1.1868	0.9272	0.3746	2.4751	0.4040	1.0785	2.6695
69	1.2043	0.9336	0.3584	2.6051	0.3839	1.0711	2.7904
70	1.2217	0.9397	0.3420	2.7475	0.3640	1.0642	2.9238
71	1.2392	0.9455	0.3256	2.9042	0.3443	1.0576	3.0716
72	1.2566	0.9511	0.3090	3.0777	0.3249	1.0515	3.2361
73	1.2741	0.9563	0.2924	3.2709	0.3057	1.0457	3.4203
74	1.2915	0.9613	0.2756	3.4874	0.2867	1.0403	3.6280
75	1.309	0.9659	0.2588	3.7321	0.2679	1.0353	3.8637
76	1.3265	0.9703	0.2419	4.0108	0.2493	1.0306	4.1336
77	1.3439	0.9744	0.2250	4.3315	0.2309	1.0263	4.4454
78	1.3614	0.9781	0.2079	4.7046	0.2126	1.0223	4.8097
79	1.3788	0.9816	0.1908	5.1446	0.1944	1.0187	5.2408
80	1.3963	0.9848	0.1736	5.6713	0.1763	1.0154	5.7588
81	1.4137	0.9877	0.1564	6.3138	0.1584	1.0125	6.3925
82	1.4312	0.9903	0.1392	7.1154	0.1405	1.0098	7.1853
83	1.4486	0.9925	0.1219	8.1443	0.1228	1.0075	8.2055
84	1.4661	0.9945	0.1045	9.5144	0.1051	1.0055	9.5668
85	1.4835	0.9962	0.0872	11.4301	0.0875	1.0038	11.4737
86	1.501	0.9976	0.0698	14.3007	0.0699	1.0024	14.3356
87	1.5184	0.9986	0.0523	19.0811	0.0524	1.0014	19.1073
88	1.5359	0.9994	0.0349	28.6363	0.0349	1.0006	28.6537
89	1.5533	0.9998	0.0175	57.2900	0.0175	1.0002	57.2987
90	1.5708	1.0000	0.0000		0.0000	1.0000	

CONCISE DICTIONARIES
(संक्षिप्त शब्दकोश)

English-English Dictionaries

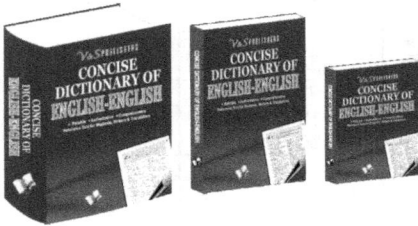

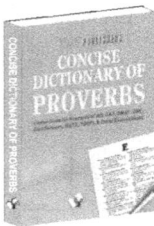

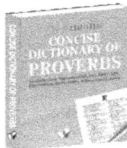

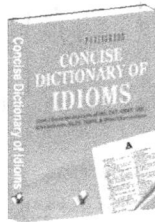

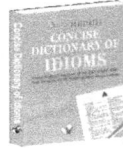

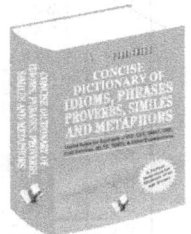

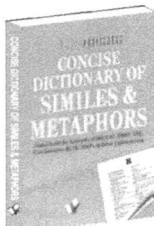

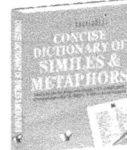

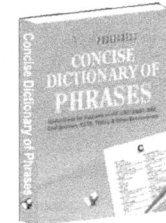

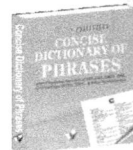

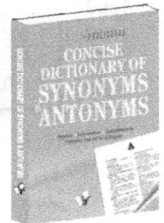

English-English-Hindi Dictionaries

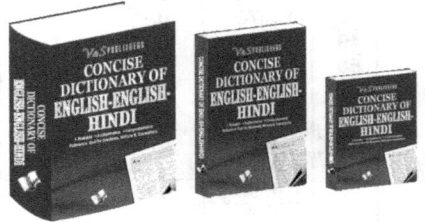

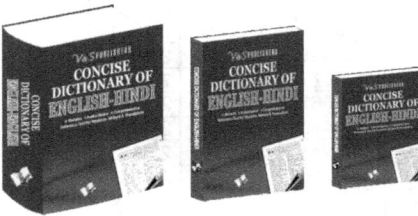

English-Hindi Dictionaries

Hindi-English Dictionaries

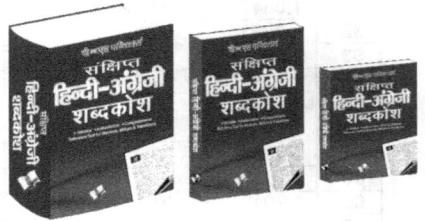

ENGLISH DICTIONARIES

All books available at www.vspublishers.com

ACADEMIC BOOKS
(शैक्षिक पुस्तकें)

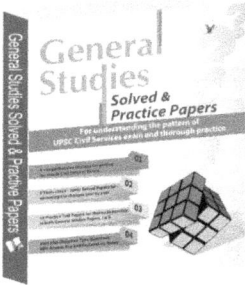

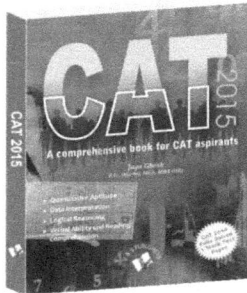

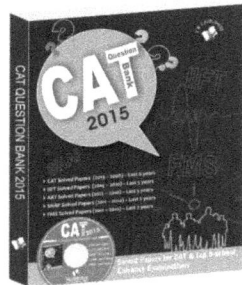

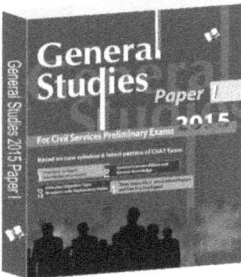

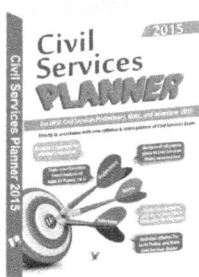

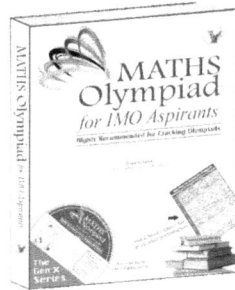

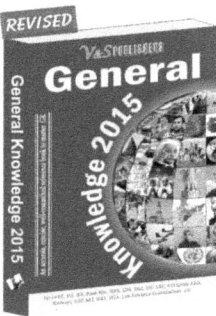

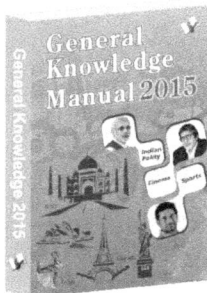

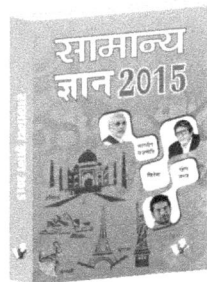

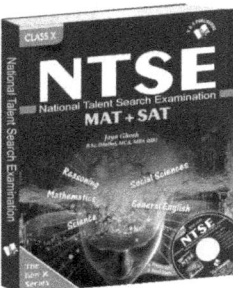

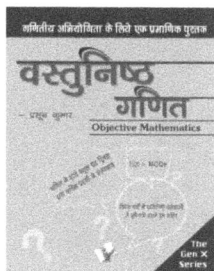

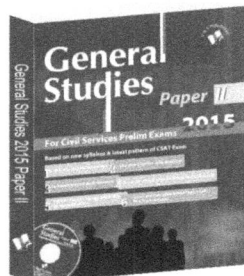

General Studies Solved & Practice Papers

General Studies Solved & Practice Papers
For understanding the pattern of UPSC Civil Services exam and thorough practice

CAT 2015
A comprehensive book for CAT aspirants
- Quantitative Aptitude
- Data Interpretation
- Logical Reasoning
- Verbal Ability and Reading Comprehension

CAT QUESTION BANK 2015
CAT Question Bank 2015

General Studies 2015 Paper I

General Studies Paper I 2015
For Civil Services Preliminary Exams
Based on new syllabus & latest pattern of CSAT Exam

Civil Services Planner 2015

Civil Services PLANNER 2015
For UPSC Civil Services Preliminary, Main, and Interview 2015

MATHS Olympiad for IMO Aspirants

MATHS Olympiad for IMO Aspirants
Highly Recommended for Cracking Olympiads
The Gen X Series

REVISED
General Knowledge 2015

V&S PUBLISHERS
General Knowledge 2015

General Knowledge 2015

General Knowledge Manual 2015

सामान्य ज्ञान 2015

CLASS X

National Talent Search Examination

NTSE
National Talent Search Examination
MAT + SAT
Jaya Ghosh
Reasoning
Social Sciences
Mathematics
Science
General English
The Gen X Series

गणितीय अभिरुचिता के लिए एक प्रामाणिक पुस्तक
वस्तुनिष्ठ गणित
Objective Mathematics
The Gen X Series

General Studies 2015 Paper II

General Studies Paper II 2015
For Civil Services Prelim Exams
Based on new syllabus & latest pattern of CSAT Exam

www.ingramcontent.com/pod-product-compliance
Lightning Source LLC
Chambersburg PA
CBHW070354270326
41926CB00014B/2544